On Being a Veterinarian

Book 2:

Getting the Most Out of Vet School

April Kung, DVM

Content disclaimer: Any incidents recounted in this series that are based on true occurrences have had select details altered to protect confidentiality. Suggestions made are based on the author's personal experience and research. Author claims no professional training or education in psychiatry, psychology, human nutrition, exercise physiology, or medical education. Please consult a certified or licensed expert in these areas for professional help. Any advice on veterinary medical practice provided by the author is intended for application by licensed veterinarians capable of using their own medical judgment. Do not attempt to use any medical advice provided by the author without a medical degree. In no event should the author be responsible or liable, directly or indirectly, for any damage or loss caused or alleged to be caused by, or in connection with, the use of or reliance on any such information provided by the author. Health-related topics, legal and financial information provided by the author should not be substituted for professional medical, legal and financial advice. It is your responsibility to research the accuracy, completeness and usefulness of all opinions and other information provided by the author. The author assumes no responsibility or liability for any consequence resulting, directly or indirectly, for any action or inaction taken based on or made in reliance on the information provided.

Published by Happy Animal Productions
First Edition December 2017
ISBN-13: 978-1-948356-01-5

This book is dedicated to the Virginia-Maryland Regional College of Veterinary Medicine Class of 2011: You will always be a part of me.

Table of Contents

Preface

Before reading this or any of the other books in this series, please download and read the free *Book Series Introduction* from my website. It explains the aim and scope of the *On Being a Veterinarian Series*, including who the series is for, and perhaps more importantly, who it's not for. Additional help and advice for future veterinarians is available on my website at www.realize.vet

In this second book in the *On Being a Veterinarian Series,* I'm going to tell you what I wish I'd known before vet school, as well as what I learned the hard way in vet school. My goal is to prepare you to get more out of veterinary school than I did (and to experience less stress along the way). As with all the books in this series, I'm speaking from the perspective of a small animal veterinarian, and my advice is likely to be most relevant to people who wish to become small animal veterinarians. This book is the most technical of the entire series and is written especially for veterinary students, or those who have been accepted to veterinary school and will be beginning their medical studies in the near future. If veterinary school is in the more distant future for you, you'll gain the most if you read this book with the intention of coming back to it again when you're about to begin vet school.

The structure of this book will closely follow the chronology of a traditional veterinary school curriculum. Obviously there exist variations between the curricula of different schools but, by and large, the macro-structure of their curricula are similar. I divide the entire curriculum into three unequal intervals based on the following descriptions:

1. The first two years of veterinary school consist of the "preclinical curriculum," where students learn basic medical science in a lecture based format. Courses in the first two years cover broad topics such as anatomy, bacteriology, virology, and medical biochemistry.
2. Year three courses, while still lecture based, are generally more focused on teaching clinically relevant medical concepts that will be directly useful in the practice of medicine.
3. The fourth year in veterinary school consists of clinical rotations, when students are meant to begin practicing medicine in a hospital setting under the guidance of experienced doctors. Each

clinical rotation typically focuses on a different medical discipline, such as radiology, surgery or neurology.

Each of these three intervals have unique characteristics and challenges. This book is going to drill down into each interval at a technical level. My goal is to forewarn you of the major challenges you should expect to face during each interval, and to provide you with concrete, proactive measures you can take to minimize stress and maximize benefits as you face those challenges.

In his Pulitzer Prize winning novel about a medical doctor practicing in Haiti, Tracy Kidder references a Haitian proverb which roughly translates to, "Beyond the mountains, there are mountains." This is an apt description for the journey you're embarking upon if you want to be a veterinarian. So, before we climb this first mountain together, I'm going to tell you a short story, and then I'm going to ask you a question. Your answer to this question might shed sufficient light on the path ahead for you to decide whether this is truly the right road for you.

Epiphany by the Park

I remember the moment I seriously considered ending my quest to become a veterinarian. I was living in Richmond, Virginia, and attending undergraduate classes at Virginia Commonwealth University. Another semester's final exams were approaching. I was sleep deprived and anxious. There was a rock in the pit of my stomach. I was riding my bike past Byrd Park on my way home from class. It was a sunny, late spring day. Water was cascading out of the fountain at the center of the park's pond, and I could hear laughter from people riding paddle boats on the water. I desperately wanted to stop my bike and sit on a park bench to watch the resident ducks swim and quack, but I couldn't. I had an organic chemistry exam to take in less than a week. I had too much studying to do.

Memories flashed through my mind of the carefree hours I used to spend walking the trails that circled that pond and wound their way around the adjacent Swan and Shields Lakes. I remembered long, leisurely conversations with friends over coffee and croissants at the French bistro a few blocks away. I fondly recalled visits to the art museum with my elderly neighbor, Dan, and how afterwards we would discuss art and life while sipping tea in his bonsai garden. How abruptly all that ended once I decided I wanted to be a veterinarian! In an instant, everything flowery and lighthearted fell out of my life, and I was transformed into a different person. All my thoughts, time and energy became laser focused on the goal of getting into vet school.

But why? Why was I sacrificing all the things that made me happy? Why was I doing this to myself? Was it my love for animals? I thought of my very first best friend from my childhood. Her name was Jackie. She was a long-haired, brown and white mutt and she let me sleep with my head on the soft fur of her belly. She never retaliated or withdrew her love when I pulled her ears or tail. When my parents argued and I was afraid, I would crawl under the dining room table, put my arms around her and feel safe again. More than thirty years later, I still feel her in my heart.

I'd been touched as deeply by every dog I'd known in the intervening decades. My kinship with them instilled in me a sensitivity to all animals, especially those covered in fur. Helping animals had always been my deepest desire. By the time I'd applied to veterinary school, I'd already spent years volunteering in animal advocacy work. Becoming a veterinarian seemed the logical next step.

As I peddled past Byrd Park that day though, the

accumulated stress of powering through multiple semesters of demanding science prerequisites had taken a toll. The thought suddenly occurred to me that I didn't have to become a veterinarian in order to help animals. I'd just been offered a full-time position with an animal advocacy organization whose mission resonated with me deeply. I could go on helping animals by taking that job, and all the burdensome worry over exams and grades and getting into vet school could be over. I could go back to the flowery and lighthearted life I had before. I could stop peddling right now and sit on that park bench.

While I rolled this tantalizing option around in my mind, I experienced a momentary lightness as every academic worry that had been weighing me down took flight and, like a flock of starlings, danced in undulating ribbons over my head, begging to be released to the wind. That was the moment I knew something else was driving me to pursue a DVM. Tempted as I was, I plucked each worry from the sky until their full weight again rested on my shoulders. Then I leaned into the wind and kept peddling. When I got home, I assumed the usual position at my study desk and began reviewing carboxylic acid derivatives for the upcoming organic chemistry exam.

I'm amazed how competing and incredibly complex trains of thought can travel our neural pathways simultaneously, and at such speed, that in a fraction of a second we can thoroughly know a thing. Yet to explain the thing in words can barely be accomplished in multiple pages of text. The following thoughts, the thoughts that prevented me from pulling the plug on my dream of becoming a veterinary doctor, proclaimed themselves in less time than it took for my bicycle wheel to complete a single revolution. Perhaps these thoughts had been mulling about in my subconscious mind for some time, and it was only the emotional turbulence of badly wanting to quit that brought them to the surface. In any case, I made up my mind in a millisecond.

The previous semester, my cat, Opy, had become very ill. He was lethargic, he wouldn't eat and he was breathing more rapidly than normal. I drove him to the emergency animal hospital where I worked as a veterinary assistant. Radiographs showed he had an enlarged heart and fluid in his chest. Three emergency veterinarians agreed: It was either cancer or heart failure. Euthanasia was recommended.

Everyone thinks their pets are special, but here's why Opy was special to me. He got his name by stepping on my keyboard and making the letters O-P-Y appear on my screen, while staring purposefully into my eyes. He made friends with the initially skittish and hostile cat living next door and brought him home, convincing him to enter our house through our dog door, despite the four dogs in residence. Opy meowed whenever I sneezed, as if to say, "Gazuntite!" Most cats will purr when you pet them, but Opy would purr even as he gazed lovingly at me from across a room.

I couldn't euthanize him without first asking my friend, Dr. Campbell, a veterinarian at a local day practice, if there were any other possible explanations other than cancer or heart failure. Truly, I expected Dr. Campbell to concur with the other three veterinarians. I was only asking to ensure I would suffer no guilty regrets after I euthanized Opy.

"Did they tap his chest?" Dr. Campbell asked me over the phone.

"No," I answered.

"Tell them to tap his chest," he said. "And tell them to look at what comes out of his chest under a microscope."

I asked the ER veterinarians to perform these procedures. They removed almost 400 milliliters of fluid from Opy's chest. What they saw under the microscope indicated Opy had a bacterial infection, not cancer and not heart failure. After two weeks of antibiotics, Opy was back to purring at me from across the room. If it hadn't been for that one doctor out of the four I'd consulted, I would have euthanized Opy for something that two weeks of antibiotics would have cured.

Before this incident, it had never occurred to me that doctors were not all equal, nor that three doctors could all agree and still be wrong. That's when I started thinking about my mother's doctors. My mother had been diagnosed with Rheumatoid Arthritis when I was young. It's a disease where the immune system gets confused and attacks the tissues of the joints as if they were a threatening invader. As far back as I can remember, my mother suffered chronic and progressively worsening pain and deteriorating mobility. Our kitchen counter was full of medication bottles. She must have been on a dozen different medicines, and it seemed, she had a different doctor appointment every week. Despite all the medications and doctor appointments though, the joints of her fingers continued to swell and her hands became more and more deformed until she could barely hold a pencil or a fork. Before she turned 50, she needed a cane to walk, and when I put my hand on her shoulder to steady her as she took one short, tentative step after another, I could feel vibrations emanating from her body as if all her joints were filled with gravel.

Up until that time, I'd taken for granted that my mother's doctors knew what they were doing. But did they? I could never hope to know without attaining a medical degree. Some things we can teach ourselves, if we're diligent; the history of the Civil War, how to play the guitar, how to start a business. But medicine is not one of those things. Only earning an MD, DO or DVM would enable me to truly understand medicine. Becoming an MD or DO would require me to practice on people, and medically speaking, I think people are gross. A DVM, on the other hand, would give me the knowledge I craved but also enable me to continue helping animals.

After landing his ships on the Yucatan peninsula in the early 16th century, Hernando Cortez knew the odds of defeating the Aztecs were slim. His troops were badly outnumbered and exhausted from the harrowing voyage across the Atlantic. Legend has it Cortez ordered his troops to burn all the ships. He created an all-or-nothing scenario. Retreat was no longer an option. Win or die. Cortez's troops won. Historians may debate whether the destruction of Cortez's ships was the deciding factor in his victory, but the story is a powerful metaphor to anyone attempting to achieve something difficult.

After my epiphany by the park, I could no longer entertain the idea of retreat. I had become fully cognizant of my primary, driving objective: The attainment of knowledge. I wanted to know what doctors know. And unlike my desire to help animals, there were no alternative paths. I burned my ships that day and, with a tenacity I previously lacked, watched the ashes of all flowery and lighthearted things drift away. I was going to become a doctor, or die trying.

That winter, during my interview at the Virginia-Maryland Regional College of Veterinary Medicine (VMRCVM) while discussing my years of animal advocacy work, I told the interviewers I hoped to continue doing that work after becoming a veterinarian. One of the interviewers asked, "If that's what you want to do, then why not just do it? Why do you need to become a veterinarian?" I replied with the clarity granted me that day on my bicycle. "What I do to help animals is for the animals, but the DVM degree is for me."

What's Your Why?

Why you want something is much more powerful than *what* you want. If you have a good enough *why,* it can get you through even the toughest times. Since you're reading this book, it's safe to assume that *what* you want is to become a veterinarian. But here is quite possibly the most important question anyone will ever ask you, and you owe it to yourself to answer honestly: *Why* do you want to be a veterinarian?

If your only reason for pursuing a DVM is that you love and want to help animals, you might want to consider alternative professions. There are other, arguably even better ways to help animals that don't require years of strenuous and expensive schooling. For some ideas on how you can help animals without becoming a veterinarian, visit www.realize.vet/book2-resources

A love for animals is an important quality for a future veterinary doctor, but in and of itself, it may not be enough to fuel you over the mountains, and the mountains beyond those mountains you must climb to become a competent clinician. Learning medicine is an arduous endeavor, and the grueling years you'll spend in veterinary school are just the beginning. Practicing medicine is even harder. To be a good veterinarian, you'll need to perpetually drive yourself to continue studying after veterinary school and throughout your entire career, even when there's no one to push you or test you.

If a passion for learning and a love of science and medicine are not among your top reasons for pursuing a DVM, you may not feel the sacrifices you make, and the effort, time, and money you spend, are worth what you gain in the end. I know it's hard to believe right now, but there's always a chance you won't like practicing small animal medicine. It happens. The great thing about the DVM degree is that there are a lot of other fulfilling things you can do with it besides clinical practice – but only if you love science and medicine.

Veterinary School: The First Two Years

There's so much I need to tell you about the first two years of vet school, and I will. But I really must begin with this: If I could go back in time and do only one thing differently, I would change the way I learned anatomy.

Study Anatomy Like a Surgeon, Not an Anatomist.

Virtually all small animal veterinarians perform surgery, whether these surgeries are elective such as ovariohysterectomies, or emergency surgeries like splenectomies or corrections of gastric dilatation volvulus (aka bloat). When you're the doctor, and no one is there to help or guide you, there is nothing more terrifying in the world than performing surgery. After you slice through skin, fat and the fibrous linea alba, there before you, sliding to and fro with every anesthetized breath, will be your patient's glistening and vulnerable abdominal organs. Now you must plunge your gloved hands inside to squeeze and pull and palpate. I promise you, unless you prepare as I suggest, the moment you, as the doctor, stand gowned, gloved and masked over your patient's open abdominal cavity, will be the moment you realize your knowledge of surgical anatomy is quite inadequate to the task.

You'll begin studying anatomy in your first semester of veterinary school. The way you'll be taught anatomy is great - if you want to be an anatomist - but it will not make you a competent surgeon. This isn't to say anatomy classes and labs won't be helpful at all. There's much to be gained from dissecting an animal cadaver down to the bones in order to memorize the minutiae of every bone, muscle, organ, artery, vein, nerve, and lymph node. But the knowledge gained from this exercise is not directly pertinent to surgery, and you won't have another opportunity later in vet school to use an animal cadaver to learn surgical anatomy.

Take advantage of your access to a real animal cadaver to teach yourself surgical anatomy as a first year student. Find out what surgical textbook your school uses and purchase or borrow one. Read the step-by-step directions for the surgeries in the following list that most small animal veterinarians need to be able to perform. Use any spare time you have in your anatomy labs to practice identifying and manipulating the tissues described until you have an understanding of the surgical procedure and a tactile familiarity with the relevant anatomical structures.

This will also help you identify gaps in your understanding of the text book descriptions. Surgical text books are written by people who know what they're doing for people who don't know what they're doing. When you know what you're doing, it's really hard to remember what it was like before you knew what you were doing. I find surgical text books sometimes skip steps that seem obvious to the experienced surgeon. If you can discover in advance what confuses you about these surgeries, you'll know which questions to ask in your surgical lectures and labs later.

- Ovariohysterectomy
- Neuter
- Cryptorchid surgery
- Umbilical hernia repair
- C-section
- Cystotomy
- Nephrectomy
- Gastrotomy
- Gastric dilatation volvulus (GDV) correction
- Gastropexy
- Enterotomy
- Small intestinal resection and anastomosis
- Splenectomy
- Diaphragmatic Hernia Repair

- Enucleation
- Lateral Suture Stabilization (for cruciate rupture in the knee)
- Limb amputations
- Laceration repair

Many of the animal cadavers we had in our anatomy labs had already been neutered or spayed. If you face the same situation, learning to identify and handle structures related to reproductive surgeries may not be possible in lab. However, you can still cross reference surgical and anatomy textbooks with your cadaver to identify where these reproductive structures were before they were excised.

During your scheduled anatomy laboratories, your professors will have their own agendas, and you may lack the time to focus on anatomy as it relates to the above surgical procedures. However, you should be able to access your anatomy cadaver outside of scheduled labs. At my vet school, first year students could use cadavers for self-directed study whenever desired as long as one of the lab rooms were free. When you begin your anatomy labs in veterinary school, ask the laboratory technicians when and how to access your cadaver outside of the scheduled labs.

If you're bold, I also suggest you ask permission to use your anatomy cadaver outside of lab time to practice skin sutures. I had to practice skin sutures on sponges as a third year veterinary student. Believe me, practicing on actual skin is a far superior learning experience. If your professor will allow this, he or she will likely give you some direction as to where on your cadaver you can practice suturing without interfering with the anatomical structures you will be studying.

Your dissection kit should contain the instruments you will need for suture practice: Scalpel, forceps, scissors, and hemostats. (Hemostats can be used during practice in lieu of proper needle holders.) You'll also need suture material. Most veterinary hospitals keep expired suture material on hand for students to practice with. Ask one of the hospital surgeons or a surgical resident if they can get you a few packs. You can also purchase practice suture online. Go to www.realize.vet/book2-resources for links.

Your surgical textbook will have descriptions and diagrams of various suture patterns, as well as instructions on proper surgical instrument handling. Read carefully, and while you practice, make sure to adhere closely to your text's recommendations on handling the instruments to avoid developing bad habits that will be hard to break later. The most important suture patterns to practice are the simple interrupted, the simple continuous, the cruciate, and the Lembert patterns. Practice tying good square knots, and burying knots under the dermis. Again, the surgical textbook will have directions to help you.

Also ask your anatomy professor if you can cut out a few small patches of skin so you can practice closing irregular defects. Unlike merely suturing closed a straight skin incision, as you would after completing an abdominal surgery, learning to close an irregular skin defect will mimic the challenges you'll face later as a veterinarian when you perform skin mass excisions, biopsies and laceration repairs. Those surgeries are not typically terrifying, but they can be frustrating and nerve racking when you find yourself unable to get the skin edges to line up without creating unsightly bulges. Your surgical text book will have directions and diagrams for closing irregular skin defects, likely in the section about skin biopsies and skin tumor removal.

If your anatomy professor won't allow you to practice suturing on your cadaver, it's most likely because they worry you'll develop incorrect technique from practicing without direct supervision, and they don't want to make the surgery professor's job harder in the future. Don't take it personally. We don't always get what we want when we ask, but if we don't ask, we never get what we want!

The Pre-Clinical Years: Huh?!

I remember how excited I was the first day of veterinary school. 7:56AM. I was sitting erect in my chair, just left of center, third row from the front, tapping my heels on the floor in nervous anticipation. I wore on my face the kind of childlike, euphoric expression you'd expect to see in a sci-fi fan about to watch the new Star Wars movie for the first time. My classmates and I had spent the first week of veterinary school participating in orientation activities. We performed trust building exercises to get to know each other better. We took the

Myers-Briggs personality test to get to know ourselves better. Now, feeling a little more comfortable in our new environment, we were ready for vet school to begin.

After conquering the abstractions of college physics and college chemistry, where, for no discernible reason, we memorized the formulae for angular acceleration and learned how to write balanced equations for various chemical reactions, finally, we had earned the right to attend lectures that would teach us something tangible and practical: How to be doctors. The clock on the wall at the front of the lecture hall ticked the final seconds down to 8AM as the first professor took the stage. All was about to be revealed.

Slowly it dawned on us that something must be wrong. Weeks went by, yet these vet school lectures seemed no different from those of our undergraduate science prerequisite courses - like biochemistry, where the only students who could possibly benefit from having to memorize the structure of all twenty-one eukaryotic amino acids were future biochemists. I remember my undergrad biochemistry professor telling me that his daughter was an MD. He'd asked her once whether what she'd learned in her undergraduate biochemistry class was useful to her as a practitioner. Her answer: "Nope. Not even a little."

Yet, even though, like my biochemistry professor's daughter and others before us, we had paid our dues by mastering the ability to draw the tyrosine amino acid molecule on demand, here we were in veterinary school where each onerous slide projected onto the screen in front of us contained the same types of abstruse diagrams we thought we'd seen the last of - diagrams populated with words like phosphoglycerate kinase, enolase and PEP carboxykinase. Even Anatomy class, with a course title that seemed to promise pearls of practical wisdom, disappointed. Instead of learning how to fix a broken leg, we memorized names for every bump, line and groove of the humerus bone. Supratrochlear foramens, lateral supracondylar crests and tricipital lines, oh my!

This is why they call the first two years of veterinary school "preclinical." It's when they teach you everything they think you need to know *before* they start teaching you how to be a doctor. It will feel a lot like your undergraduate science courses except for two important things: The quantity of information you're going to be expected to digest, and the time you're going to be given to digest it.

As an undergrad, I had two to four lectures per day, three to four days a week. I had ample time to read and ponder to develop a robust appreciation of the material, as well as the smug satisfaction of knowing I could correctly answer any exam question my professor could ask. Even though as an undergraduate student I had to push myself very hard in the week or two before mid-term and final exams, afterwards there was plenty of time to recuperate. After mid-terms, I had half a semester before final exams. After final exams, there was a long holiday or summer break before the next semester began.

In vet school, classes ran Monday through Friday from 8AM until 5 or 6PM, with one hour for lunch – though often there were lectures to attend during lunch as well. When I got home at night, I had six to eight minutes to feed and talk to my dogs while I waited for my microwave dinner to cook. Then I practiced the art of blindly scooping food onto a fork and maneuvering that fork to my mouth while my eyes reviewed the material that was covered in school that day.

After about the first month, it seemed there was at least one exam a week. Preparing for the next exam was my constant and only priority. Whatever the focus of next examination, it took precedence above all else. I had little choice but to neglect my studies in every other subject because I knew, despite my best efforts, I wouldn't be able to answer every exam question correctly. And never, in the first two years of vet school, did I ever feel I had developed "a robust appreciation" for any of the material. No matter how much I studied, I was always behind. There was always a book chapter or a set of lecture notes or a journal article I needed to read but couldn't get to before the exam. After the exam, there was no time to revisit those neglected materials, gems of medical wisdom though they might have contained. The stopwatch for the race to the next exam had already started ticking.

I longed to take a few days off from classes just to catch up on sleep and reading, but this was out of the question. Class attendance was mandatory. Excused absences for illness were possible to attain, but due to the mountains of material covered every day, they would be academically impossible to make up. Hence, throughout the seasons the classroom was filled with the sounds of sniffling, sneezing, nose blowing, and coughing. The sounds of sickness grew noticeably more severe right before an exam. I kept a scarf with me to cover my nose and mouth each time a nearby classmate coughed or sneezed, so I rarely got sick. I did, however, spend the entire first four semesters struggling to stay awake in a dark lecture hall despite never getting enough sleep, and doing my best to sit erect despite the progressively worsening, pulling pain in the strained muscles of my neck. People can talk all they want about the importance of maintaining good posture when you sit at a desk, but let them study medical biochemistry and embryology every night of the week until 2AM and let's see if they don't slouch.

To try to alleviate my neck pain, I bought a contraption off the internet that consisted of a metal hanger that you were supposed to affix to the top of a door. It had a pulley, and a rope that fed through the pulley. On one end of the rope there was a hat-like apparatus with a chin strap, and on the other end of the rope there was a handle. Nightly, I put my head in the hat-like apparatus and pulled the handle to momentarily relieve the muscles of my neck of the burden of supporting my head. I don't know if it helped or not.

Semester after semester, professor after professor took to the stage at the front of the lecture hall to present another seemingly endless parade of random, complicated factoids that I would do my best to memorize. Never was it made clear how all these factoids were related to each other, or how they related to the practice of medicine. One first year professor did warn us that we would feel like someone stuck a fire hose in our mouths and turned the water up all the way. But, since at the time, I expected this promised geyser of information to be delivered with some semblance of rhyme and reason, my initial response to his warning was, 'Bring it!'

In actuality, it felt more like a high-powered pitching machine was aimed at us, but instead of shooting baseballs, it spewed millions of tiny puzzle pieces like confetti over our heads, every minute, all day long. Our job was to catch every tiny, precious piece. But there were so many. It wasn't possible to catch them all. Which ones were most important? We didn't know. And where to put them when we caught them? No one had shown us the puzzle box cover so we didn't know how to arrange them.

I'm not telling you this to dishearten or frighten you. If you love science, fascination will pull you through. If you fit the mold of the stereotypical veterinary student, your achievement-oriented nature will find some kind of masochistic enjoyment in rising to these challenges. I merely want you to be prepared so that when you arrive at this juncture in your educational journey, unlike me, you'll waste no time or energy feeling confused, shocked or frustrated. And in the following sections, I'll give you some practical advice for dealing with the two biggest challenges of the preclinical years.

Challenge #1: Too Many Puzzle Pieces

I've known people who failed their first or second year of vet school, not because they weren't smart enough, but because they were overwhelmed by the sheer quantity of information being spewed at them. It was more than that though. We were all overwhelmed. The people who failed were the ones who became psychologically overwhelmed at the thought of being academically overwhelmed. That's what did them in. Here are some tips to help you avoid that.

Don't try to be the best

I got a 95% on my first undergrad organic chemistry exam. When I learned the class average was under 50%, I felt oh so very smug. Perhaps I shouldn't admit this, but the truth is, I absolutely loved that feeling. As an undergrad, the competitive drive to always get the highest grade in the class was my turbo boost. Achieving that objective gave me a huge, egotistical dopamine rush.

It became immediately apparent however, once I started vet school, that I was no longer the smartest person in the room. Perhaps you will be the smartest person in your veterinary class, but chances are, like me, you'll find yourself surrounded by people who are just as smart as you, if not smarter. But don't despair. Look at it this way: If you find that you're average in a room full of super smart people, congratulate yourself! That's awesome!

Don't waste your energy trying to compete with your vet school classmates. They may catch puzzle pieces you miss, but instead of competing with them, learn to collaborate with them instead. When you start your career as a veterinarian, being a skillful collaborator will be of far greater value than being the best at catching every random factoid puzzle piece out of the air just so you can get the highest score on an exam.

Don't think you're the worst

Suddenly finding yourself surrounded by very smart people in an unfamiliar environment may unnerve and intimidate you. You might wonder if some mistake was made in your school's selection process. You may find yourself thinking that everyone in the class is better and smarter than you, and that you really don't belong there. You might worry that someone will eventually figure it out, and you'll be asked to leave. You'll tell yourself that your success so far has been due to luck, or charm, or even the fact that you work really, *really* hard.[2,11] After all, if you were legitimately intelligent, you wouldn't have had to work so hard to get an A in organic chemistry.

If you allow thoughts like this to fester in your mind they will lead to anxiety, and potentially, depression.[11] You're going to have enough to deal with as a new veterinary student without taking on this additional and unnecessary psychological burden. If these soul sucking thoughts start whispering in your ear, recognize them for what they are: normal but irrational, and quite common in high achievers.[2] They are a part of a phenomenon first described by two psychologists in 1978 and most commonly referred to as Imposter Syndrome. Luckily for my class, our first year professors talked openly about this and assured us that, despite our secret fears and insecurities, we had indeed been thoroughly vetted. They promised we had been accepted into this competitive program based on our merits, and every one of us deserved to be there.

Knowing it exists and feeling comfortable speaking openly about it are two of the most powerful weapons against Imposter Syndrome. If you experience Imposter Syndrome and no one else talks about it when you begin veterinary school, speak with a professional. Some veterinary colleges have on-site counselors who should be very familiar with this energy sucking monster. If your vet school doesn't have counselors for vet students, make it a priority to find a therapist yourself.

Above all, remember this: Success is the culmination of persistent determination combined with competence over many years. If you get into vet school, it will be because you demonstrated persistent determination and competence for a long, long time. Suddenly finding yourself surrounded by very smart people in an unfamiliar environment doesn't invalidate your previous successes. It is a result of those successes.

Let go of perfectionism

Just as high achievers are more prone to experiencing Imposter Syndrome, they're also more likely to be perfectionists. This isn't a coincidence. Perfectionism and

Imposter Syndrome are like two different ends of a mad dog chasing his own tail. High achievers often attribute their success to their perfectionism. They drive themselves to produce a perfect result, and repeated success achieved in this manner eventually leads them to believe that perfectionism is the source of their success. When perfectionists fall short of perfection, as they inevitably do, they drive themselves even harder. Over time, they develop an unconscious belief that "their successes must be due to that self-torture,"[11] rather than innate ability. This is how the seed of Imposter Syndrome gets planted.

Despite your perfectionist tendencies (and despite the very real and valid qualifications that will actually get you into vet school), the outlandish number of puzzle pieces you're going to be responsible for, combined with the inadequate time you'll be given to catch them all, are going to cause you to fall far shorter of your own expectations than ever before. You will fail to complete every reading assignment. You will not achieve perfect understanding of the material. You will answer questions in class incorrectly. You will answer questions on exams incorrectly. You will not get an A in every class. Some semesters, you may not get an A in any class.

Try to remember that you're in the upper echelons of academia. It's supposed to be hard. Give yourself permission to be an imperfect human being who sometimes needs to sleep instead of study. Give yourself permission to merely pass a class (gasp!) instead of acing it. Give yourself permission to do the best you can without torturing yourself, and see what happens. I bet you'll realize you're good enough without having to be perfect.

And if you fail? It's not the end of the world. It's most likely not even the end of vet school! The students in my class who failed were given an opportunity to try again the following year. Most of them took that opportunity and went on to graduate as Doctors of Veterinary Medicine. When you begin vet school, find out what your school's policy is on this matter. My guess is, unless you get kicked out for cheating or some other bad behavior, you'll be given another chance. So relax! Even if you're not perfect, you're unlikely to fail, and even if you fail, you can try again!

After an exam, forget the exam

The stress before taking an exam is intense. The stress after taking an exam and waiting to find out if you passed may be just as bad. You don't need that extra stress. Sometimes you'll wait hours for the test results, sometimes days. It's hard to concentrate on anything else while you're wondering if you've just bombed out of vet school. To prevent this prolonged post-test anxiety, before handing my test in, I'd count every one of my answers that I thought could be wrong – any answer I wasn't 100% certain of. Then I'd subtract the number of suspect answers by the total number of test questions, and divide that number by the total number of questions. For instance, if I was uncertain about 12 answers and the test had a total of 50 questions, $50 - 12 = 38$. $38 / 50 =$

0.76 or 76%. Therefore, I could be reasonably sure I got at least a 76% on that test, which is a passing grade. After the exam, while my classmates vibrated with anxiety as they talked with each other in the hallway about who answered what to which question, I'd go buy a cup of tea from the cafeteria and relax until the next lecture started.

Usually, my exam score ended up being higher than my calculated worst-case scenario. Very rarely, it was lower, but only by a percentage point or two. Doing this calculation before you hand in your exam can give you the peace of mind to forget the exam and focus on other things until the scores are posted.

Maintain your health

When my mother first saw me after two semesters of organic chemistry, she was very upset about how much weight I'd gained. She was not the type of person who cared about superficial things. She wasn't upset because of how she thought my physical appearance would reflect on her. She was worried about the psychological effects it would have on me when I started vet school. "You're going to feel very insecure about yourself and that's going to make everything harder on you," she said, her forehead wrinkled with worry and loving concern.

Vet school is going to feel a lot like high school. In the beginning, there will be that uncomfortable period of not knowing anyone and having to make new friends. My mother was right. My weight did make me feel insecure, and that made me reluctant to socialize with new people.

The first several months were especially tough, because not only did I feel like an imposter, I felt like a lonely, overweight imposter. Even my face was chubby. I couldn't hide that under oversized sweaters.

Four years is a long time to be seeing the same classmates and professors every day. I guess it was natural that I developed a few crushes along the way. Perhaps you'll end up developing little crushes too. My weight caused me even more distress every time I had to see one of those crushes. The worst part was having to wear scrubs for some of our labs. Scrubs are about the least flattering kind of clothing there is, but on top of that, the scrubs we ordered had different colored drawstrings depending on their size. Small sizes had pink drawstrings, medium sizes had beige drawstrings, and large sizes had white drawstrings. I needed a large. I was mortified at the thought of having to advertise my scrub size to my crush, so before labs started, I went to the drug store and bought fabric dye. I dyed my white drawstrings beige. You don't need this extra stress in vet school!

I hope by the time you start vet school you'll have taken my advice from Book 1 and you'll already have gotten yourself in good physical condition. It's much easier to maintain physical fitness than it is to attain it. I couldn't lose weight while in vet school, but if I'd been fit when I started, I could have maintained physical fitness. So, ideally, get fit before vet school, and then commit to maintaining.

The rigors of the first two years are going to make you feel like you have to put your own health on the back-burner in order to get through. After all, when you're in class Monday through Friday for eight to nine hours a day, and studying every night and weekend, something's got to give. But that something should not be you. You will actually do better academically if your body stays fit, and you will certainly do better psychologically.

The human mind is robust enough to allow for self-protecting mechanisms in pursuit of a goal. So tell your brain that you want it to get you successfully through vet school without sacrificing your physical or psychological health. Review my suggestions from Book 1 and design a minimum weekly exercise regimen. Maybe get up thirty minutes early and do fifteen minutes of high-intensity interval training (HIIT) and 15 minutes of yoga before classes.

Find a study group

Discussing material with other students will enhance your understanding. Other people will catch puzzle pieces you missed. You'll have caught pieces they missed. You may have different ways of interpreting some of the pieces. By sharing and discussing, each member of the study group will benefit from an enhanced perspective that none could have attained alone. This is synergy. My recommendation is that study groups contain between three and six people. Fewer than three and synergy is diminished. Greater than six and chaos ensues.

In my veterinary class, many study groups formed,

disbanded and formed again with different members in the first year. This is normal. People were searching for others with whom they could feel comfortable. This takes time and experimentation. It's important that you feel comfortable with the people in your study group because, in order to learn new things, you'll need to admit when you don't understand something, and you won't be willing to show this vulnerability unless you feel rapport with others in your group.

Lastly, and perhaps much more importantly, because there is so precious little free time, vet school study groups provide essential social support. Solitary study is necessary and it's how you'll probably spend most of your time, but studying with other people on a regular basis will drastically reduce your stress level. You'll be able to laugh and commiserate and remember that you're a human being.

My fondest memories and deepest friendships from veterinary school came from the people in my study group. I couldn't have made it through without their help and encouragement. I'm eternally grateful to them, and expect we'll be friends to the end of our days. My wish is for you to find an equally wonderful group of classmates to accompany you through this incredibly challenging but rewarding period of your life.

Record every lecture

You would be amazed how little you actually remember (or even hear) when you're madly scribbling (or typing) notes for eight or nine hours a day. Obviously you won't have time to re-listen to every lecture, but when you begin studying in earnest for an exam, I guarantee you'll come across concepts you'd initially perceived as straightforward but turn out, on further scrutiny, to be positively confounding. In those instances, you'll be very glad to have the option of re-listening to the lecture. There were occasions I had to re-listen to sections of a lecture three or four times before I felt I truly understood a concept.

Get into the habit of naming and uploading the day's lectures to your computer the moment you get home every evening. It may sound like an onerous task to have to perform every night after a long, hard day of classes, but it really only takes a few minutes. If you wait a week or two before performing this task, you'll have forty-five to a hundred recordings to cross check against each day's schedule before you can correctly name and file them.

Here's how I kept all my lecture recordings organized. I created computer folders with the following hierarchy: First level folders were labeled by vet school year. Second level folders were labeled by semester. Third level folders were labeled by course name.

Every evening, using the day's lecture schedule, I matched each of the days' recordings based on their chronological order in my recorder, and used the day's corresponding class notes to name each recording with the course name, date and topic (for example, *Neuro 11-2-09 – Seizures*). To this day, I have audio files of all of my veterinary school lectures. On occasions when I've wanted to review a specific topic, it's been easy to find the lecture I needed. Below is a modified screenshot from my computer to illustrate.

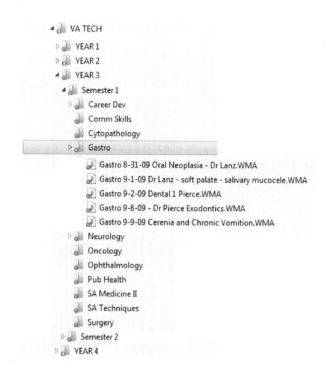

Challenge #2: Half the Puzzle Pieces are for the Wrong Puzzle

Most of the classes in the first two years of veterinary school are taught by academic veterinarians or academic physicians (board certified specialists who do not practice) or PhDs (or PhD-DVMs or PhD-MDs) who are specialists in their fields but do not practice medicine. The same can be said for human medical schools. PhDs, academic physicians and academic veterinarians who spend their days immersed in research see the world through a very different lens than practicing medical doctors. Although efforts are being made to make preclinical science courses more clinically relevant, since the professors are not clinicians, much of the information is bound to be either clinically irrelevant or presented in a way that obscures its clinical relevance.

This isn't to say everything you'll learn in your first two years of vet school is unnecessary, but you should expect to feel much like the nineteenth century store merchant John Wannamaker when he complained, "Half the money I spend on advertising is wasted; the trouble is I don't know which half." Similarly, about half the puzzle pieces spewed at you during your first two years of veterinary school will not be relevant to you as a future practitioner. You just won't know which half.

Does a future veterinarian really need to learn the entire life cycle of multiple types of parasitic intestinal coccidia? Yes, he does. Does a future veterinarian really need to learn every step and factor in the cascade of molecular events that leads to a blood clot? She does indeed. Does a veterinarian really need to memorize the molecular structure of the steroid hydrocortisone or to know whether an injectable antibiotic is an acid or a base in order to practice medicine? No, and heck no.

Don't get me wrong. My pre-clinical professors were brilliant and eminently likable people. The warm memories I have of them remain with me still. Each of them had the students' best interests at heart and wanted to help us become successful professionals. Even though not everything I learned from them was clinically relevant, much of it was still amazing and interesting. It's just that many of the puzzle pieces I got from them were for the wrong puzzle – like the puzzle for becoming a research scientist, instead of the puzzle for being a clinician.

Why is it like this? Because pre-clinical professors, just like veterinary students in the pre-clinical years, have to operate within a pre-existing medical academic system that has been evolving slowly and imperfectly for over a century. Today's medical curricula are descended from the model of medical education created by very smart and dedicated people over a hundred years ago.[4] Before they came along, if you were studying medicine in the United States, you would likely have been attending a private, for-profit school with little in the way of entrance requirements aside from your ability to pay tuition. There was no regulation and no standardization to guarantee the quality of medical education and training.

Then, in the early twentieth century, medical education in the United States underwent a major overhaul. A group of progressive scientists and educators, including the founding dean of the John Hopkins University, coalesced around the goal of standardizing medical education on a solid foundation of science and research. Following the example of German universities, and with financial help from philanthropic grants from sources such as the Rockefeller Foundation, medical faculty were freed from any direct patient care responsibilities, and employed full-time in research and teaching. Their primary objective became the advancement of biomedical knowledge.[4,9]

During this period, the logic behind housing medical research and medical education under the same roof was sound. Researchers were focused on tangible medical problems such as whether diseases such as scurvy and rickets were due to nutritional deficiencies, and which brain structures were responsible for what functions. Answers to questions such as these could directly and immediately help graduating medical doctors better care for their patients. The marriage between medical research and medical education was a great boon, producing countless medical advances such as blood transfusions, pacemakers and electrocardiographs, the discovery of insulin, antibiotics, and the development of vaccines to prevent diseases like polio, diphtheria and typhus.

But pause for a moment to consider the exponential increase in scientific and medical knowledge since that time. In a 2003 article entitled *The Internal Challenges to Medical Education*, author Kenneth Ludmerer points out, "Before World War II, a notable characteristic of medical research was the relatively short distance from the standard [medical] student courses to the forefront of medical research."[8] Since that time however, astronomical progress has been made in both medical research and medical practice.

Research scientists today are splicing genes, investigating the molecular behavior of JAK inhibitors, and measuring interleukin-1 receptor antagonist concentrations. This kind of work takes decades or more to translate into clinically relevant medical knowledge. The intellectual chasm between medical researchers and medical practitioners has grown too vast to accommodate the easy communication they once enjoyed. Like two childhood sweethearts, both have grown up, and in the process, have grown apart. Ludmerer refers to this intellectual distance as a "bench-bedside gap," and asserts that it raises "profound new questions about who should teach medical students and the interrelationship of teaching and research."[8]

Though many are aware of the problem, we can't just throw out the traditional medical curriculum and start all over from scratch. The medical school infrastructure was built on the traditional curriculum. If we tear it down to build something else, where would we live in the mean time? Where would those researchers go? Would important progress in biomedical research be stalled? For how long? Where would medical colleges get the funding they need if not through research grant money? Who would teach the pre-clinical material to medical students?

This is why the preclinical years are the way they are. It's no one's fault. A lot of people in both human and veterinary medical education are trying to find solutions. Many vet schools are trying to revamp their curricula to be more clinically relevant, but they must make changes within the existing infrastructure in a way that doesn't destabilize that infrastructure. Progress can be slow.

Astrophysicist Carl Sagan wrote something in his book *Cosmos* that forever changed the way I see the world. He was explaining why the human brain isn't perfect, but I found it an apt metaphor for so many of the world's imperfections, including the imperfections of today's medical education system. He said:

"There is no way for evolution to rip out the ancient interior of the brain because of its imperfections and replace it with something of more modern manufacture. The brain must function during the renovation. [...] The old parts are in charge of too many fundamental functions for them to be replaced altogether. So they wheeze along, out-of-date and sometimes counterproductive, but a necessary consequence of our evolution."

So, while you can't avoid having to memorize clinically irrelevant material in veterinary school, (relevant to your future as a doctor or not, you're still going to get asked about it on exams), I can help you better recognize which puzzle pieces are likely to be clinically relevant. Then I'll provide different strategies for learning the pieces you'll need as a doctor versus memorizing the pieces you'll only need to pass your exams. Let's start with the big picture.

The Puzzle Box Cover
for the Future Clinician

Most sources will define the practice of medicine as the science of preventing, diagnosing and treating disease. I think this is an apt definition unless you're studying to become a doctor. For medical students, this definition falls short. It contains no hint as to *how* a medical doctor prevents, diagnoses and treats disease. Just try solving for x in the following equation:

Doctor + x = ± prevention ± diagnosis ± treatment

What is x?

The standard definition for the practice of medicine doesn't provide adequate information to solve this equation. Most people will intuit that x represents some kind of specialized knowledge, but what is the nature of that knowledge? Some might say x represents knowledge of the body, and that would be correct, but still too vague for someone who endeavors to obtain that knowledge. I suggest you think of the practice of medicine as applying one's **knowledge of the structure and function of body systems to prevent, diagnose and treat disease**. This is the puzzle box cover for the future clinician.

What is a body system? It's a collection of organs and tissues that work in concert to perform specific functions necessary for life. For example, the cardiovascular system includes the heart and all the blood vessels in the body. The cardiovascular body system performs the function of delivering oxygenated blood and clearing metabolic cellular waste such as carbon dioxide to and from every cell in the body. Basic knowledge of this body system would include knowing the macro and molecular structure of the heart, understanding how it functions as a whole organ, and how its different parts function individually and together.

You would also need to know what electrical, biochemical and hormonal impulses affect it, as well as the structure and function of arteries, veins and capillary vessels, and what mechanical, chemical and hormonal impulses affect them. Additionally, you would need to understand how the heart and vascular system work together, as well as all the things that can go wrong, why they go wrong, and how they go wrong.

Here's a list of the main body systems for your reference:

- Cardiovascular system
- Respiratory system
- Nervous system
- Sensory systems
- Musculoskeletal system

- Digestive system
- Urinary system
- Reproductive system
- Endocrine system
- Hemolympathic system
- Integumentary system

To illustrate why knowledge of body systems is fundamental to learning, and ultimately, to practicing medicine, imagine yourself as a veterinarian working in a small animal clinic. A sick dog is presented to you. What are the first two things you need to do?

1. Perform a physical exam
2. Get a thorough patient history from the owner

Why? Because the information you get from the exam and history tells you which body systems are most likely affected. If an owner tells you her dog is reluctant to get out of bed and you find knee pain on your physical exam, you would look closer at the musculoskeletal system. If an owner tells you her dog has been coughing and you also notice the patient is having some trouble breathing, the respiratory system is one of the body systems you should further investigate.

Once you determine which body systems are involved, everything else will follow, including which diagnostic tests to order. Even if your initial test results don't provide a definitive diagnosis, knowing which body systems are affected may still help you formulate a reasonable treatment plan, if the owner isn't willing or able to pursue additional testing.

This seems obvious in hindsight. Yet, it wasn't until halfway through my second year of vet school that I was finally able to infer that knowledge of the structure and function of body systems to prevent, diagnose and treat disease was the puzzle box cover I needed to make sense of what I was being taught. I consider myself a reasonably intelligent person, so why did it take me so long to figure out? Why did my classmates and I suffer through hours, days, weeks, and months of lectures feeling so perplexed, and wondering when we were going to learn to be doctors instead of factoid memorizing, test taking automatons?

It's because, in addition to half the puzzle pieces being for the wrong puzzle, the pre-clinical curriculum is discipline focused, rather than body system focused. Logistically, it makes sense to do it this way since the majority of pre-clinical veterinary school professors specialize in research disciplines, not body systems.[3] So virology was taught by a virologist, pharmacology by a pharmacologist, toxicology by a toxicologist, and so on. Even many of the more clinically relevant courses were taught by doctors who specialized in disciplines such as radiology or pathology.

Clinically relevant information in the pre-clinical years is like the character of Osiris in the Egyptian myth. Osiris was the giver of life and the god of the cycles of life. He represented proper order in the universe. But he was murdered by his brother, who shredded his body and scattered the tiny pieces all over Egypt. In a discipline-based medical curriculum, the body system puzzle pieces are scattered throughout different discipline-based courses. These courses *do* teach about body systems, but they teach about them in fragments, and only as they relate to each discipline.

In histopathology class, one day we could be taught how to use a microscope to identify red blood cells (the hemolympathic system). Later that day, in embryology class, perhaps we'd learn about how the placenta develops during gestation in different species (the reproductive system). After that, in physiology class, we might get to hear about all the molecular interactions that occur during muscle contractions (the musculoskeletal system).

In order to get the most out of your first two years of veterinary school, you're going to need to be like Isis, the sister of Osiris, who searched for and reassembled the fragments of Osiris's body. You'll have to search for the fragments of body systems knowledge, and assemble them onto your own mental scaffold with the goal of increasing your understanding of body systems one tiny puzzle piece at a time.

As your understanding of body systems grows, you'll get better at recognizing the clinically relevant material. You'll notice that every course will, at times, describe how their subject matter relates to certain body systems in terms of preventing, diagnosing and treating disease in those systems. For example, regardless of which parasite you may be studying in your Parasitology class, you'll learn which body systems the organism is most likely to affect during different parts of its life cycle. In your Bacteriology class, you'll learn about how different bacteria tend to infect certain body systems more than others, and when you study Oncology, you'll learn that different types of cancers also have a tendency to arise in particular body systems.

To help you recognize when you're being taught something you need to know as a veterinarian (such as why calcium is crucial for muscle contractions or which antibiotics are harmful to the kidneys) versus what you only need to know long enough to pass an exam (such as every molecular step in the G-protein cell signaling cascade), continually ask yourself: **Is this something that could enhance my knowledge of the structure and function of body systems for the purpose of preventing, diagnosing or treating disease?** Another way to discern whether material is clinically relevant is if the professor delivering the lecture is a practicing clinician in the teaching hospital. If she is, she's most likely going to talk about things that are relevant to medical practitioners. I can't guarantee you'll get it right every time, but with the body systems puzzle box cover you'll do a better job of distinguishing what's really important in your first two years than I was able to.

Learning What You Need Versus Memorizing What You Must

Part of me wishes I could go back and repeat the first two years of vet school knowing what I know now. I have the feeling I missed a lot of clinical gems before figuring out the difference between puzzle pieces for the clinician puzzle and puzzle pieces for the research scientist puzzle. I just used rote memorization for every piece I could catch. When there are too many puzzle pieces, and you can't see the big picture, rote memorization is what you use to pass exams. But rote memorization isn't ideal for building the kind of knowledge base that will be useful when you start practicing.

Knowing what you know now, you can better distinguish between what you need to learn versus what you must merely memorize. Study for long-term retention anything that looks like it will enhance your understanding of body systems and the prevention, diagnosis and treatment of disease. Use rote memorization for the rest.

Learning what you need

Socrates said that learning is remembering. He didn't mean it the way I mean it here, but I'm using his quote to make a point. If you really learn something, you remember it forever. Even if the details get fuzzy with time, the information remains in your brain and can be revived with minimal effort. Your goal is to learn clinically relevant information, so you'll want to study those puzzle pieces with the goal of getting them into your long-term memory. One way of doing this is to associate new information with other facts that are already in your long-term memory. This is called "meaningful learning," because you store new ideas in a way that has meaning for you. When I talk about adding clinically relevant puzzle pieces to your mental scaffold, this is what I mean.

If you've known anyone whose dog was being treated for heartworm disease, or if you've worked at a clinic where a patient was being treated for it, you probably know that after a dog is given injections to kill the worms, the dog's physical activity must be severely restricted for the next two months. He can't run, play or physically exert himself in any way. This you already know. It's a part of your long-term memory and you'll never forget it (barring neurological degeneration).

When you begin to learn the pathophysiology of heartworm disease in veterinary school, two important facts you'll want to remember are:

1. These worms are most likely to be found in the pulmonary artery (the artery that leads from the right side of the heart to the lungs).
2. One potential complication of heartworm disease is pulmonary embolism, which is a blockage of smaller branch pulmonary arteries by fragments of heartworms that have been killed by the injections the veterinarian gave. A pulmonary embolism prevents blood from circulating through the lungs, picking up oxygen

and carrying that oxygen to the rest of the body. This can be debilitating, painful and even fatal. The harder and faster the heart of a dog with heartworm disease pumps, the more likely fragments of dead heartworms will cause pulmonary emboli. This is why activity restriction is essential after heartworm killing injections have been given.

If you connect the above new information to what you already knew, you're unlikely to forget where heartworms are usually found in a dog, and that one potential complication of treating heartworm disease is pulmonary embolism. Once these new facts become part of your long-term memory, they too can be used to help you remember other important things, such as the anatomical structure of the heart, the vessels leading into and out of the heart, and how blood flows through the heart and those vessels. Just like a spider spinning a web, the more connections you create to and between your long-term memories, the larger and more resilient the entire structure becomes.

You can create elaborate drawings to help you learn things in a meaningful way, too. Buy some markers and a few pads of easel paper measuring 23" x 32" and draw the heart and everything related to the cardiovascular system on one page. Do the same for the urinary system, and the digestive system. Add to your drawings as the semesters progress and as your understanding grows. Here's a picture of a 23" x 32" drawing I made as a first year veterinary student. Don't try to discern the details of the picture. It's been radically reduced to fit on this page. I provide it only in case you're interested in a visual idea of what these drawings may look like.

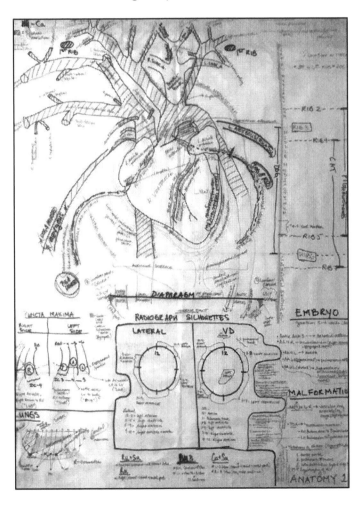

You can also use mnemonics, which are basically just made up associations you create to help you remember. Mnemonics can be used for short-term and long-term memory, but they're one of my favorite long-term memory tricks. Generally speaking, the more meaningful a mnemonic is, and the simpler it is, the more likely it is to stick in your long-term memory.

Here's an example of a meaningful mnemonic that can aid long-term memory: Two terms you'll learn in vet school that you should remember because they pertain to the diagnosis of disease are "sensitivity" and "specificity." In the context of medicine, these terms are used to quantify how good a diagnostic test is, such as the heartworm test. How good a test is depends on how often it's right or wrong. A diagnostic test can be right in two ways, and it can be wrong in two ways.

A test can be right when it says the patient has a disease and the patient has the disease. This is called a "true positive." It can also be right when it says the patient doesn't have a disease and the patient doesn't have the disease. This is called a "true negative." A test can be wrong when it says the patient has a disease but the patient doesn't have the disease. This is called a "false positive." And a test can be wrong when it says the patient doesn't have a disease but the patient does have the disease. This is called a "false negative." A test that yields a high percentage of true positives is said to have a high specificity. A test that yields a high percentage of true negatives is said to have a high sensitivity. A test that yields a lot of false positives has a low specificity, and a test that yields a lot of false negatives has a low sensitivity.

Do you have a headache yet? If you tried to memorize that, it would be time consuming and unlikely to stay in your long-term memory. It's too complicated! We need a short-cut. So here's the mnemonic I devised to remember what I needed: The word "specificity" has the letter **P** in it, and "s**P**ecificity" relates to true and false **P**ositives. The word "sensitivity" has the letter **N** in it, and "se**N**sitivity" relates to true and false **N**egatives. Then, just like exam scores, high is better than low, so a test with high specificity is better than a test with low specificity. High s**P**ecificity means it yields a lot of true **P**ositives and few false **P**ositives, so I'm more likely to believe a **P**ositive result from a test with high s**P**ecificity. A test with high sensitivity is better than a test with low sensitivity. High se**N**sitivity means it yields a high number of true **N**egatives and few false **N**egatives, so I'm more likely to believe a **N**egative result from a test with high se**N**sitivity. Now if someone tells me a test has a specificity of 95% and a sensitivity of 93%, I can feel pretty confident about the results of that test, be they positive or negative. If someone tells me a test has a specificity of 60% and a sensitivity of 70%, maybe I need to take the positive and negative results of that test with a grain of salt and compare them with more scrutiny against clinical signs and other test results, as well as how common that disease actually is.

What if a test has 95% s**P**ecificity and 40% se**N**sitivity?

Is it a good test? How about a test with 40% sPecificity and 95% seNsitivity? Is that a good test? It depends on whether you want to rule-IN a disease (confirm your suspicion the patient has the disease), or rule-OUT a disease (confirm your suspicion the patient does not have the disease). If you want to rule-IN a disease, you need a test with a high number of true Positives – so a test with high sPecificity is a good test for ruling-IN a disease. If you want to rule-OUT a disease, you need a test that yields a lot of true Negatives – so a test with a high seNsitivity is a good test for ruling-OUT a disease.

The mnemonic I use to remember the association between rule-IN and high sPecificity tests versus rule-OUT and high SeNsitivity tests is, if I rule-IN a disease, I can tell the pet owner very sPecifically what disease we're dealing with and what sPecifically we need to do about it. If I rule-OUT a disease, I need to be seNsitive about the way I explain this to a pet owner. It's frustrating to pay for a test and have the doctor tell you the result is negative, because now you've spent a bunch of money but you don't have an answer. For that pet owner, I'd need to use seNsitivity to explain that ruling-OUT a disease does provide useful information because it means we can focus our attention on more likely explanations for what's wrong with their pet.

Memorizing what you must

Rote memorization is simple repetition. It can be used for long-term memory. This is how most of us learned the alphabet and our multiplication tables. But I've found rote memorization especially helpful when I needed to memorize large amounts of information in a short period of time *without* needing to understand it or remember it forever. I used rote memorization to help me pass my final exam in bacteriology.

The exam was taking place the next day, and was going to cover fifty-six different organisms. For each organism, I was supposed to know what shape they were, what species of animal they were most likely to infect, what part of the body they usually infected, what physical signs they were likely to produce, what complications could arise, whether there was a vaccine for that organism, whether they were gram negative or positive, oxidase positive or negative (this relates to a laboratory test where bacteria turn a culture medium a different color depending on whether they produce a certain enzyme), whether they were motile or not (another criteria used in the laboratory to help identify an organism), whether they were strict aerobes (needing oxygen), strict anaerobes (thriving only in the absence of oxygen), whether they would prefer an absence of oxygen but could tolerate oxygen, whether they could tolerate a lot or only a little oxygen, whether they lived on the inside of an animal's cells (intracellular) or outside the cells (extracellular), whether they had capsules or not, whether they produced gas or not, whether animals infected with them could be "carriers" (meaning the animal is not symptomatic but still able to infect other animals), whether they could be "vectored" (transmitted to infect other animals by some other organism, like mosquitoes or ticks), whether or not they were a part of an animal's normal flora (like a population of bacteria that normally live in an animal's digestive system and typically cause no harm), and whether or not they were "zoonotic" (being transmissible between humans and other animals).

When you're in lecture learning about these different types of bacteria, and you're maybe covering five or six a day, it all seems perfectly manageable. Of course you'll be able to remember them! One was an anaerobe, the other was a strict aerobe, two were zoonotic, and one was intracellular. Easy! But the night before the exam, you realize that details that seemed easy to remember are not so easy at all when you have to remember them for fifty-six organisms.

I tried for hours to study all the details in a meaningful way, but it was no use. There were way too many puzzle pieces. At around midnight, I started to panic. Nothing was sticking in my brain. I was going to fail my final exam in bacteriology and get kicked out of vet school. That's when I decided to use rote memorization. I created a chart. It was a complicated chart, but it condensed and simplified everything I had to remember. I listed each organism and then I created symbols for all the different characteristics. I drew the appropriate symbols next to the name of each organism. And then, I memorized the whole bloody chart. I forced myself to recreate that chart on a blank piece of paper over and over and over again until I could do it perfectly. And then I did it one more time before going to bed at 3AM, and three more times the next morning when I woke up at 6AM. During the exam, I simply sketched that chart on the question sheet and referred to it as I answered each question.

Ideal? No. Necessary sometimes? Yes. As a clinician, was it necessary for me to really learn all of those details? No. Some of them, but not all. As a matter of fact, not even most! But, I passed that exam, and now when I need to find detailed information on specific bacteria, I look it up in a book! I used charts like that for pharmacology and parasitology. And I used rote memorization diagrams for anatomy – such as when I had to memorize all the branches of the mesenteric arteries. Just for kicks, on the following page is a picture the chart I created for my bacteriology final exam. Again, don't try to make out the details. I include it only for your entertainment.

40

G- / Oxidase+ Rods	Fam Anaplasmataceae (ENA)
Pasteurellaceae (AH)	**Ehrlichia (REC)**
Actinobacillus spp.	Ehrlichia ruminatum
Haemophilus spp.	Ehrlichia ewingii
Spiral/Curved (HALC)	Ehrlichia canis
Heliobacter spp.	**Neorickettsia (HER)**
	Neorickettsia helminthoeca, elokominica
Lawsonia intracellularis	Neorickettsia risticii
Campylobacter spp.	**Anaplasma (MP₂)**
Spirochetes (BLBT)	Anaplasma marginale
Borrelia burgdorferi	Anaplasma phagocytophilum
Leptospira interrogans serovar pomona	Anaplasma platys
Brachyspira hyodysenteriae	**Fam Rickettsiaceae (RC)**
Treponema brennaborense	Rickettsia rickettsii
Ncategory Strict Aerobes (BBM)	Coxiella Burnetii
Bordatella bronchisepta	**Fam Chlamydiaceae (FAP₂)**
Brucella spp.	Chlamydophila felis
Moraxella bovis	Chlamydophila abortus
Pseudomonas aeroginosa	Chlamydophila pecorum
NSF Anaerobes	Chlamydophila psittaci
Mycoplasms (18)	**FUNGI**
Mycoplasma cyanos, canis	**Superficial/Cutaneous (MC-M₂T)**
Mycoplasma felis	Malassezia pachydermatitis
Mycoplasma hyorhinis, hyosynoviae, hyopneumonia	Candida albicans
Mycoplasma gallisepticum, synoviae, meleagridis, iowae	**Dermatophytes**
	Microsporum canis
Mycoplasma capricolum, ovipneumoniae, conjunctivae	Microsporum nanum
Mycoplasma mycoides ss mycoides	Trichophyton mentagrophytes
Mycoplasma bovis, californicum, canadense	**Intermediate / Subcutaneous (MS)**
	Mycetoma (7 spp: BACLAPE)
Mycoplasma bovigenitalium	Sporothrix schenckii
Hemotro-Mycoplasms (SH₂OW)	**Deep/Systemic (BHC₂C₂)**
Mycoplasma suis	Blastomyces dermatitidis
Mycoplasma haemocanis	Histoplasma capsulatum
Mycoplasma haemofelis	Coccidioides immitis, posadasii
Mycoplasma ovis	Cryptococcus neoformas, gatii
Mycoplasma wenyonni	**Miscelaneous / Opportunistic (ZA)**
Ureaplasms (DC₂F)	Zygomycosis (6 orders, 800 species)
Ureaplasm diversum	Aspergillus spp.
Ureaplasm canigenitalium	**PRIONS**
Ureaplasm cati, felinum	

✱ = Intracellular
C = capsule/asteroid body
d = dimorphic (Fungi imperfecti)
Z = zoonotic
g = gas production

= Strict aerobe
= strict anaerobe
= microaerophilic
= aerotolerant
= susceptibility test

M = motile
N = normal flora
⊙ = carrier state

These are just a few of my favorite tricks for both long-term retention and short-term memorization. There are many books available that focus on various study methodologies that you can refer to for additional tactics. Before you start veterinary school, I recommend you peruse a few of them to collect a handful of different tips and tricks that will work best for you. Just remember - the key is to use study tactics for long-term retention for information related to body systems and disease prevention, diagnosis and treatment, and short-term memorization tactics for the rest.

Some may be scandalized by the suggestion that vet students who want to be practicing small animal veterinarians should concentrate their efforts on material they identify as more clinically relevant, and only pseudo-memorize the rest. Well, the undeniable reality of the first two years of veterinary school is that there are too many puzzle pieces! No human being, no matter how smart or hard working, can catch every one of them. I'm just giving you the advantage of being better able to discern which puzzle pieces are more likely to be relevant to your future as a clinician, and which aren't. If you get it wrong and label something unimportant that's actually important, take comfort in knowing two things: First, even factoids you use rote memorization for can stick in your brain for a long time. Second, the important stuff is always reiterated throughout the four years – so if you miss it (or diss it) the first time, you'll get it the second time, or the third time, or the fourth time.

Year Three: Thinking Like a Doctor

I remember one first year professor's comforting words to my friends and me as we studied for an embryology exam. She was about to begin her lecture when she noticed we'd spent the ten minute break before her class struggling to memorize every word in a complicated illustration of extraembryonic membranes. She assured us it wouldn't always feel so impossible and overwhelming. She said we would eventually start thinking like doctors, and then everything would get easier. But, I wanted to ask, how will I know when that happens? What will it feel like? What if it doesn't happen?! Can you give me an approximate date as to when this will happen so if it doesn't happen by that date I can... I don't know... Do something?

I'll forever remember the kindness that professor extended to us that day, but I'll be honest – I didn't believe her. "You'll eventually start thinking like doctors." What does that even mean? It sounded just like promises I'd heard for spiritual enlightenment. Just keep working at it, and someday, I don't know when, I don't know where, and I don't how... But someday, a bright ray of light will beam down on you from the heavens and a chorus of angels will sing your name.

But you know what? That professor's promise did come true. I was halfway through the second semester of my second year. I was slumped in my chair in a darkened lecture hall, listening to a talk about anemia in clinical pathology. My professor was providing a case history for a patient that had been treated at our teaching hospital. I was scribbling copious notes as usual, trying to capture every word, when all at once something shifted in my brain. It was like all the information I'd been presented up to that moment was as senseless as a pile of iron filings, and then someone turned on an electromagnet and order emerged. I felt like Dr. McCoy in the original Star Trek episode, *Spock's Brain,* after he puts an alien civilization's "teaching machine" on his head and everything suddenly becomes clear. "It's so simple," Dr. McCoy exclaims, "a child could do it!"

I stopped writing, sat up straight, took a deep breath, and sighed with relief. It was the first time I ever truly relaxed in veterinary school. Before that moment, the stress of trying to catch every single puzzle piece was crushing and unrelenting. But instantly, somehow I knew, I would continue to pass exams without having to memorize every infinitesimal detail. A metamorphosis had occurred.

Once I was blind, but now I could see! The scales had been removed from my eyes! The big picture! There it was, right in front of my face! I understood which puzzle pieces mattered and how they fit together. I had started to think like a doctor, and I didn't need to fret anymore about exams because now I could reason my way to the answers!

When you start thinking like a doctor, it's nothing short of a *"Eureka!"* moment. All your sacrifices and hard work will seem worth it, and you'll dance and strut from one subject to the next, eager to apply your new powers of understanding and to quench your thirst for more medical knowledge. You'll be as Tantalus standing in the pool of water that had always receded before he could drink, and under the fruit trees whose branches always blew out of his reach before he could grab their fruit – except on the day you begin thinking like a doctor – the water will not recede and the fruit will not be out of reach. You will be free to consume as much as you can stand.

I don't know for certain what causes this transform-ation. I don't know if the process of information overload combined with being under great mental and physical strain for long periods is what causes it. I don't know if it's taking specific medical courses in a specific order, or if it's one particular course alone that causes the transformation. I can tell you that not everyone experiences this transformation as an instantaneous epiphany. My husband recalls that for him it occurred later (during his internship year) and much more gradually.

But whether sudden or gradual, this metamorphosis marks an important milestone in the education of every medical doctor, whether human or veterinary. It's when the door of a previously impenetrable fortress swings open, and all the wisdom of the ages is there for the taking. Though you are not yet a doctor when it happens, your neural pathways have been sufficiently primed for medical knowledge to take hold, because you can finally see from a clinical perspective.

It would seem the admission fee to pass through this door is the persistent banging of one's head against it for a period of time which varies by individual. Based on my observations of my classmates and of myself, the transformation seems to happen for most vet students at some point between the second semester of second year and the end of the first semester of the third year. The transformation may happen later for students in MD and DO programs because the curricula between veterinary schools and human medical schools diverge after the second year.

MD and DO students start their clinical rotations in their third year of medical school. Based on my conversations with my husband, it seems they may start clinics before they're able to understand what they're seeing. By contrast, veterinary students get the luxury of one more year of didactic, classroom learning. Some might think having to sit all day, every day in classroom for another year sounds awful, but this is a year very unlike the previous two years.

Year three in veterinary school is taught almost exclusively by practicing clinicians from the teaching hospital, which means, virtually everything you'll learn in year three will be clinically relevant. Is it any surprise then that most veterinary students start thinking like doctors during this period? While I admit I don't know what causes this wonderful transformation to take place, I suspect it has a lot to do with how quickly you're able to able to develop a robust mental scaffold of all the body systems. I think the moment you start to think like a doctor is the moment you start to see the connections between all the body systems.

Completing the Clinician Puzzle

When we set our minds to accomplishing something enormous and complex, such as a completing a puzzle with millions of pieces for example, we start by assembling smaller, more manageable sections. Only after many of those smaller sections have been completed can we start to see how they fit together. Using the body systems scaffold during your first two years of veterinary school should help you assemble many large sections of the clinician puzzle. Year three of vet school is when you start connecting those sections to complete the puzzle.

No longer a slave to manic memorization, and not yet

an indentured servant to the responsibilities of clinical rotations, your third year of veterinary school is when you'll have the freedom of the luxury of extra time and energy. Put this freedom to good use. Start building conceptual bridges between all the different body systems to understand how they work together and how pathology in one affects the others. Then, since by this point you'll be able to make sense of material presented in a discipline-based format, you can start connecting body systems and medical disciplines, such as those related to disease prevention (e.g., nutrition, vaccinology), disease diagnosis (e.g., radiology, clinical pathology, histopathology) and disease treatment (e.g., pharmacology, surgery).

While learning about the role the liver plays in drug metabolism, go back to your anatomy notes and study the portal venous system, noticing how the entire venous vasculature of the gastrointestinal tract drains to the liver. What difference does this make if you're thinking about giving a drug orally versus intravenously? While you're learning about interpreting radiographs or ultrasonographic images of the abdomen, consult your notes on the reproductive system and figure out how to use imaging to diagnose a pyometra. While studying the pelvic limb in your musculoskeletal class, use your surgical textbook to cross-reference your musculoskeletal class notes against the surgical procedures for a femoral head ostectomy (FHO) and the tibial plateau leveling osteostomy (TPLO). When you're learning about cardiology, look into how a sick heart might affect the kidneys, and how sick kidneys might affect the heart. How might the relationship between heart and kidneys complicate treatment in a patient with both heart and kidney disease? While you're learning about pancreatitis in dogs and cats, review the structure of the duodenum in your anatomy notes to figure out why cats (and people) with pancreatitis end up with sick livers more commonly than dogs with pancreatitis.

Here's a realistic scenario to demonstrate why it's important for clinicians to have built good conceptual bridges between all the body systems and the medical disciplines used to prevent, diagnose and treat disease:

***

A patient initially presents because the owner noticed a draining wound on the dog's foot. Samples were collected and examined via cytology under a microscope but results were inconclusive. Radiographs of the digit indicated abnormalities in the bone. The veterinarian decides to perform an excisional biopsy of the toe under anesthesia. The excised toe will be sent out for a histopathological analysis and a bacterial culture. While the veterinarian is visualizing the ligaments she needs to transect, she is also planning how to close the surgical laceration in the skin. She is contemplating post-operative antibiotics. She is cognizant of the plane of anesthesia the patient is under and the type and amount of pre-induction medications that were administered. If readings on the ECG monitor change, she must interpret them to discern if the patient's heart is responding to pain impulses or if cardiovascular compromise is occurring. She is thinking about the results of the patient's pre-operative blood work and how that will affect her choice of post-operative pain medications. She is formulating a plan for how the surgical wound should be managed until it's fully healed. She is thinking about next steps if the histopathologist tells her it's cancer. She's thinking about different options to discuss with the pet owner depending on what kind of cancer...

***

We assign body systems and medical disciplines to categories because it helps us organize the information in our brains so we can learn and communicate about these topics. But the perfect delineations in our brains between these categories don't exist when we practice real medicine on real patients. Completing the clinician puzzle is about making all those straight and curvy lines between the separate puzzle pieces disappear until all we see is one seamless big picture. You won't complete the clinician puzzle in your third year of veterinary school, or in your fourth year, or even in your first year of practice. But third year is when you'll begin completing the puzzle.

Supplemental Learning

No professor, no matter how dedicated, smart or talented, can provide a perfect representation of a complex medical topic in an hour long lecture. Nor can they adequately elucidate the important clinical connections between the topic at hand and other medical subjects. They will do their best to summarize what they believe to be the essential highlights, but what they elect to omit because of time constraints may be just that critical piece of information that would have taken your understanding to a more sophisticated level. Can you pass your exams and get through veterinary school by just going to lectures and studying only the lecture notes and slides? Yes. But you're reading this book because you want to get the most out of veterinary school. Why do you want to get the most out of veterinary school? I presume it's because you want to be an amazing veterinarian. If you want to be an amazing veterinarian, you need to consult alternate sources of medical information in addition to what you learn in your classes. Following are some supplemental learning resources that can help you accelerate the process of completing the clinician puzzle.

> ***Veterinary Information Network (VIN):*** As a veterinary student, you can get free access at www.vin.com. VIN is used by many practicing veterinarians. I consider it an essential resource and personally would not practice without it. It's staffed by almost 300 veterinary specialists who monitor discussion boards on specific topics and answer questions from veterinarians. To find information on any topic, simply type your query into the search box and you'll get a list of online discussions, both past and present, related to your search query. If no one else has asked what you want to ask, you can start a new discussion. For your future reference, VIN also offers online

continuing education courses and a Classifieds section that will be helpful when you're ready to start your job search. Additionally, it has a free sister site (www.veterinarypartner.com) where I often refer my clients so they can obtain more information on specific medical conditions in plain language from a reputable source.

Journal of Veterinary Internal Medicine (JVIM): I subscribed to this journal after graduating from veterinary school. If I remember correctly, it cost me over $200 a year, but I felt it was worth it for the depth of medical explanation it provided. Lucky for you, it's free now via the Wiley Online Library. Search Google for *JVIM Wiley* and it should be the first result. Enter any query into the search field (make sure you're on the JVIM page and that "In this journal" is selected) and you'll get a list of every related article published in this journal. You can even get a JVIM app to search and read articles on your smart phone.

Journal of the American Medical Association (JAVMA): When I was a veterinary student, we were offered a discount on annual subscriptions for this journal. If you register for this journal as a veterinary student, I suggest you elect the online version only. You can only search by medical topic via an online interface anyway, and that's

going to be your primary use for this journal. It's unlikely you'll find the time to leisurely read whatever articles happen to appear in the magazine when it's mailed to you every two weeks. I made the mistake of signing up for both online access and the printed edition. By the time I finished vet school, I had a column of neatly stacked, unread JAVMA magazines as tall as I am.

Tips on using supplemental sources

When reading a journal article about a specific topic, I suggest reading only the introduction paragraphs and the *"Discussion"* section. If there is insight for a veterinary student to gain on a specific topic, it is most likely to be found in those sections and not the sections about experimental design and statistical analysis. If you decide to specialize after you earn your DVM, you'll learn more about scrutinizing those sections, but for now, I'd ignore them. Just take any conclusions in the article with a grain of salt because if the methods or analyses are suspect, the conclusion may be invalid. It's more likely that the value of these articles for you will be in their elucidation of physiological or pathophysiological mechanisms rather than specific conclusions.

If an article isn't quite on target in terms of what you're looking for, or if you want to delve deeper into something you find in the initial article, scan the reference list at the end of the article for other titles of interest. Ask the librarian in the medical library of your school whether you can freely access academic and research articles through their system. If you can, take every advantage. Obtaining full articles from intriguing titles in a reference list can yield a treasure trove of helpful and interesting information.

Some of the referenced articles you'll see in veterinary academic journals may be from journals on human medicine. In many veterinary journal articles the authors may describe what is known about the topic in human medicine because more is known as it pertains to humans. Some of the best learning I've obtained has been from human medical journals and human medical text books. In general, I've found them to provide a depth and breadth unparalleled in veterinary medical literature. This is because much more money is spent in human medicine and medical research meant to inform human medicine. I highly suggest consulting human medical journals and texts, especially if you're having difficulty with a particular concept. Just remember, despite striking physiological and anatomical similarities between humans and other mammalian species, differences do exist, and any mechanisms or treatments described should not be assumed as universally applicable. Use human medical literature to learn, not to practice.

Lastly, save any articles you find interesting or

helpful. You'll want to refer back to them as your education progresses, and once you start practicing. Save them in either paper or digital folders that are arranged according to body systems. This will make it easier to find them later.

Year Four: Practicing to Practice Medicine

At my VMRCVM interview, I was given some great advice by one of the six doctors on the panel. It was nearing the end of the meeting and after answering their questions for nearly an hour, I had been given the opportunity to question them. I asked just one thing.

"At the emergency hospital where I work," I began, "they just hired a veterinarian who is fresh out of vet school."

The members of the panel nodded, letting me know I had their attention.

"On his first day, as his first patient was carried back from the lobby for him to examine," I continued, "he stood rigid and still as a statue for almost a minute. His eyes were wide and I'm pretty sure he stopped breathing. To me, he appeared paralyzed with fear, and I felt so bad for him. I thought to myself, 'Oh dear! Four years of veterinary school and you still end up terrified on your first day.'"

Several members of the panel grunted as if to say they knew where this was headed.

"My question for each of you is," I paused for effect, "what can I do as a veterinary student so that I don't feel like that on my first day of practice?"

The one answer I received was the only answer I needed.

"Think of your clinical rotations in your fourth year of veterinary school," replied the dapper doctor in a dark blue suit on my right, "as practicing... with a net."

If it hadn't been for the impression that terrified new grad made on me, the question it planted in my mind and the resulting astute advice I received later at my interview, I would have thought of my clinical rotations as my last year of veterinary school, rather than my first year of practice. If it hadn't been for the invaluable advice the dapper doctor gave me, I would have thought of clinical rotations as merely another year of learning, instead of a year to practice applying everything I'd already learned. I wouldn't have pushed myself so hard to understand everything so thoroughly in the first three years, since I'd have expected more opportunities to learn it all again later in fourth year. And I would have spent my fourth year of veterinary school waiting to see what the real doctors decided to do, rather than asking myself what I would do if I were the doctor in charge.

Despite the great advice and how it helped me get the most out of clinical rotations, the catchy phrase the dapper doctor used isn't completely accurate. The truth is, you don't really get to practice medicine as a fourth year student. You get to watch and assist and sometimes role play with real doctors as they practice medicine, but the best you can do as a fourth year student is to practice practicing medicine. Believe me though, at this junction in your education, that's all you want.

Practicing with a net is what interns do. Interns are doctors, and they make real medical decisions about patients that are really their patients, and even though they may be working under the supervision of a more experienced clinician ("the net"), they have all the responsibilities of a real doctor – because that's what they are. I wasn't ready for that as a fourth year vet student! Heck, I wasn't even ready for that after I graduated and started practicing! But, I'll tell you what... I'd have been a lot less ready to practice if I hadn't used clinical rotations to practice practicing medicine.

I'm making this sound like a choice, and it is. You can easily look at your fourth year as another year to learn instead of a year to apply what you've already learned, though I suspect you'll choose to use it more productively now that you know you can. Of course, it's not as simple as that. It's not *just* a choice. It's also a challenge. As a fourth year veterinary student, your most important role is that of a student-doctor practicing to practice medicine. However, you'll have many other roles to play, and these other roles will be time consuming and laborious. You'll have to be proactive about practicing to practice medicine, and it won't be easy.

Your Role as Master of Scutwork

The first four to six weeks of clinical rotations is all about figuring out how the giant monstrosity of complexity called the teaching hospital actually works. There are so many different departments, and they all work together in different ways depending on what a patient needs. Dermatology calls anesthesiology when a skin mass needs to be surgically removed. Internal medicine needs radiology to perform ultrasounds, cardiology to do echocardiograms, and the hospital laboratory to run blood work. Some of the laboratory tests the doctors order can't be performed in the teaching hospital and have to be sent out to other laboratories all over the country. Neurology needs radiology to do MRIs and CT scans, and radiology needs anesthesiology to induce and monitor anesthetized patients for these procedures. Patients in the ICU need medicines from the pharmacy. Every patient enters the teaching hospital through the admissions protocols of the administrators at the front desk, and every patient record needs to be continually updated with the billing department so that when a patient is discharged, the front desk administrators can tell the pet owner what their final bill is.

Newton's third law of motion states that for every action there is an equal and opposite reaction. The veterinary teaching hospital's first law of motion is that for every action there is at least one, and more often multiple forms to fill out before any action can occur. The veterinary teaching hospital's second law is that it's the student's job to fill out those forms. (Medical students and interns in human medicine call this scutwork.) The third law is which forms need to be filled out and where those forms need to be delivered will vary depending on who the veterinary student asks.

I'm a systems person. I continually create, revise and redesign systems in order to keep my life running efficiently. I've created workflow and communications and chain-of-approval systems for previous employers. My philosophy is that a life without good systems is a life without sense. One of my definitions of hell is being part of a system I don't understand, especially an imperfect system, which I would define as one in which there are differences of opinion as to how it works. My first month in the teaching hospital was this kind of hell.

My first hospital rotation was called "Community Practice." It was supposed to give fourth year students experience in a general practice or day practice setting. Within the first few days, I had discovered the third law of the veterinary teaching hospital. If I asked three different people which forms to fill out and where to take them when I was done, I would get three different answers. This was not only frustrating but it also caused me a great deal of anxiety. I wanted to do everything right. The system I developed to compensate for the imperfections of the hospital system was to ask as many people as it took until two people both gave me identical answers.

One of the people I often asked was my dear friend Claire, who was on the rotation with me. Chloe is one of the nicest people you could ever meet. Only once, in all the time I've known her, have I ever seen her speak harshly to anyone. It was to me, on that rotation. Over the course of a couple weeks, she had witnessed me asking multiple other people the same questions I'd previously asked her. Finally, on one of these occasions, she got to see someone else provide the same answer she had. My satisfaction that I now had the right answer – apparently thanks to this other person - is probably what set her off. "What the heck?" She snapped. "I told you the exact same thing half an hour ago!"

From the first moment you first step into the teaching hospital as a fourth year veterinary student, set your mind at once to figuring out what the workflow protocols of the hospital are, who the players are in every department, and what "scutwork" you're supposed to do. In addition to figuring out which forms need to be filled out for what purposes and where they need to be delivered, you'll also need to know how far in advance the forms need to be delivered depending on what's being ordered or requested.

Every department will have its own schedule and its own ways of managing its resources. Some departments need more advance notice than others. If you fail to turn in the forms on time, a procedure your attending clinician needed to perform could be delayed. It will also be your job to run blood and tissue samples to the laboratory, and to pick up the results when they're ready so you can deliver them to your attending clinician. Ordering and retrieving medications from the pharmacy for surgeries, for hospitalized patients and for patients being discharged will also be your job.

You will feel confused, overwhelmed and frustrated as you try to learn your responsibilities as Master of Scutwork. Different people will give you different answers, and you'll get blamed for doing things incorrectly, regardless of who told you to do it that way. When a computer user wants to verify that another computer on the network is working properly, they perform what's called a "ping test." A "ping" is a data packet that's sent out and gets echoed back. Time for the echo to return and whether the returning echo is missing any information tells the user whether the system they're pinging is reliable. You're going to have do a lot of pinging when you begin clinical rotations to determine which "systems" are reliable. Do your best to remain polite, and try to retain a sense of humor as you find your way, even if other people get frustrated with you for asking too many questions or for asking someone else the same question you just asked them! Eventually, you'll learn which people in the hospital really know how things are supposed to be done, and they'll become your go-to people when you have questions. Be extra, super, duper nice to these people. Bring them cupcakes.

Your Role as a Veterinary Assistant or Technician

On most rotations, the lion's share your time will be spent on patient care as a veterinary assistant or technician, not as a student-doctor. You'll restrain patients, draw blood, place IV catheters, set up IV fluids, and perform treatments. Common treatments you'll be tasked with include administering IV and oral medications, taking and recording vitals like heart rate, respiratory rate and body temperature, icing surgical sites, performing physical therapy, wound care and bandage changes, cleaning dirty cages, and taking hospitalized dogs outside to urinate and defecate (an especially onerous task if your patient happens to be heavy and physically impaired).

In my mind, that great advice about using clinical rotations to practice practicing medicine, did not include the work I had to do as an assistant or technician. I resented that work. I never shirked my duties in directly caring for my patients, but I did everything I could to avoid restraining patients, drawing blood and placing IV catheters. My attitude was that when I became a veterinarian, those things would be someone else's job. Why should I be forced to do that work instead of spending my time practicing the more important role of student-doctor?

Here's why: When my husband wants blood drawn, or radiographs taken, or medications administered, or one of his patient's toenails clipped, he goes to his desk at the hospital, sits down in front of a computer terminal, types what he wants done on his keyboard, and then hits "Enter." His orders are transmitted by computer system to all the appropriate parties, and everything he wants done is performed by other people, in some other part of the hospital. If these other people need help drawing blood because the patient has imperfect veins, or they need assistance lifting an especially heavy patient onto an x-ray table, they do not call my husband for help. I expected my role as a veterinarian to be the same! Nope!

The reality of my role as a veterinarian is if the technicians I'm working with can't draw blood or place an IV catheter, I have to do it. If they need help lifting a patient onto the x-ray table, or if they're not sure how to position the patient for an x-ray, I have to help. If I ask someone to start fluids on a hospitalized patient, that person may not know how the fluid pump works and I will have to do it. If there is a very naughty dog in the hospital who is supposed to get his toenails clipped, I (along with three other people) will have to help restrain him.

Only in retrospect do I see the value of practicing all those veterinary assistant and technician skills in clinical rotations. I was lucky to start my career as a veterinarian in a great emergency hospital where the technicians were highly skilled, but in truth, I was only postponing my need to develop those skills by relying on those amazing ER technicians. When I transitioned to general practice, I had a very rude awakening. What do you do if even the veterinarian is unable to draw blood? What do you tell the client?

To avoid this very unpleasant situation, jump at every opportunity to draw blood and place IV catheters when you're a fourth year student. Appreciate it when you learn how to set up a fluid pump, when you learn how to tube-feed a cat, or monitor a blood transfusion, or perform coupage, or ice an incision, or perform physical therapy, or change bandages - because you will need to know how to do these things as a veterinarian – either because you'll be doing them, or because you'll need to teach someone else how to do them. If you're one of those precocious future vet students who has lots of clinical experience, and you're already good at blood draws and IV catheter placements, when you get to clinical rotations, reinforce your skills by teaching less experienced fourth year students what you know.

Your Role as a Laborer

Being a veterinary assistant or technician is hard labor. Clinical rotations are about 75% hard labor. You will assist in surgical preparation, and monitoring anesthesia during surgeries and imaging procedures like CAT scans and MRIs. Afterwards you will sit with post-op patients until they are awake enough to have their endotracheal tubes removed. On surgical rotations, you will scrub in and assist by holding instruments or internal organs as directed by the surgeon.

Some surgeons will talk you through their surgeries and quiz you on the procedures. Other surgeons, especially resident surgeons, will likely be concentrating too hard to talk while they operate. In those cases, you'll find yourself holding a pair of hemostats in the same position for hours in silence, while trying to ignore your full bladder, the itch on your nose and the cramps in your hands.

At my veterinary school, typically the most dreaded small animal rotations were orthopedic surgery, soft tissue surgery and neurology (because of neurosurgeries). The surgeries themselves often took several hours (neurology surgeries typically went on for four to six hours or more, and I even heard of one lasting twelve hours). But after those long surgeries, many taking place late at night or even in the middle of the night, the student's work would not be done. The post-surgical care for those patients is also the student's rsponsibility. One really sick soft tissue surgery patient, like a post-op cholecystectomy, could easily require four or more hours day of patient care. The same could be said for an otherwise healthy, post-operative hip replacement or back surgery patient.

On my neurology rotation, the luck of the draw had me caring for a 130 pound, obese Golden Retriever named Vincent, whose very kind and doting owners brought him Oreo cookies every day. Vincent didn't need surgery but his MRI revealed he'd suffered a cerebellar stroke. The cerebellum is one of the parts of the brain involved in balance. Poor Vincent felt like the world was spinning all the time. He couldn't walk because he was too dizzy, and if he wasn't appropriately positioned and packed between multiple mats in his hospital cage, he would incessantly roll to the right, wrapping himself up in his IV lines.

I had to perform physical therapy on Vincent twice a day. This consisted of lifting his enormous, right careening body into a sling centered inside a four wheeled structure made of metal bars. After accomplishing the herculean task of getting Vincent into this contraption, I'd be panting and red-faced. A wet, warm sheen of perspiration would break out all over my body as I adjusted the height of the sling so Vincent's feet touched the floor. Then, I had to push him up and down the hospital hallways so he could practice walking and re-learn which way was up. Vincent didn't seem to understand the purpose of these excursions. Mostly he just relaxed in the sling, let his feet drag on the smooth floors of the hospital, wagged his tail, and panted sideways, but happily, at everyone we passed. I loved Vincent and his family, but caring for him in the hospital required several hours a day, and on top of all my other duties, he wasn't the only patient I had to take care of.

Small Animal Internal Medicine rotations can also be very demanding because patients on these services are often severely ill. These are the medical cases that are too complex or too involved for most day practice veterinarians to tackle, or they're patients that continued to decline despite treatment provided by other veterinary

84

hospitals. On these rotations you may expect to see things like gastrointestinal lymphoma with virtually constant vomiting and diarrhea (guess who gets to clean that up), or a jaundiced cat with severe hepatic lipidosis requiring tube feeding every four hours, or severe bronchopneumonia requiring frequent IV antibiotics, nebulization and coupage every four to six hours.

Unless your teaching hospital has an Emergency Medicine rotation, you will probably also have to take turns with your classmates being on-call for overnight emergencies. I didn't even bother going home on the nights I was on-call because every round trip per emergency call would cost me twenty minutes of precious sleep, and I'd already been up all day performing the duties of my regular rotation. Instead, I brought a blanket, pillow and alarm clock and tried my best to get an hour or two of sleep between emergency calls in one of the hospital conference rooms. On one especially busy night, I worked for 36 hours straight. During the 34th hour of that ordeal, while trying to simultaneously eat an apple and type my medical records, I started crying like a baby wishing my mommy were there to put her arms around me.

Your Role as a Student-Doctor: Ideal Versus Real

When a new patient arrives at the teaching hospital, the fourth year veterinary student is responsible for taking a history from the pet owner (why they brought their pet to the hospital, what clinical signs the pet was exhibiting, what other medical issues the pet might have, and any medications the pet was currently taking). Then the student-doctor performs the initial physical exam. After that, the student-doctor presents to a senior clinician, intern or resident. The presentation begins with the patient's signalment, (the patient's age, sex, species, and breed – which is important because different disease processes are more or less likely depending on the signalment), followed by the history and physical exam findings.

The student-doctor's presentation would sound something like this: "This is a nine year old, female spayed American Staffordshire Terrier with a three-day history of progressively worsening lethargy and inappetence. On physical exam, she is dull but alert and responsive, icteric, tachycardic with a heart rate of 130 bpm, febrile with a rectal temperature of 104 F, and non-painful on abdominal palpation. She takes Rimadyl twice daily for mild arthritis but has no other significant medical history."

Once the student-doctor completes the presentation, the senior clinician will ask for a list of differential diagnoses (multiple possible explanations for the patient's clinical signs). In this example, some obvious differential diagnoses would be hepatitis, gall bladder mucocele, ascending cholangitis or cholangiohepatitis, and immune mediated hemolytic anemia. Based on the list of differential diagnoses, the student-doctor will then be asked to formulate a diagnostic plan for determining the actual (aka "definitive") diagnosis. A diagnostic plan dictates which tests should be performed, and in what order, to most efficiently either rule-in or rule-out different suspected diseases.

After this, the senior clinician and student-doctor will enter the exam room together and the senior clinician will clarify the patient history with the pet owner and repeat the physical exam. The list of differential diagnoses and the diagnostic plan will be modified per the senior clinician's findings and judgment. Then while the student-doctor observes, the senior clinician will explain to the pet owner what illnesses are suspected based on the clinical signs and physical exam findings, which diagnostic tests are being recommended and why, and depending on time constraints and the mood of the clinician, what the potential treatment plans might be for the most likely diagnoses.

Ideally, the student-doctor's initial presentation will take place in a quiet conference room without distractions, and the senior clinician will thoroughly analyze and gently guide the student-doctor's thought processes. When they return together to the exam room, the senior clinician will coach the student-doctor while a second physical exam is performed. Any exam findings missed or misinterpreted will be emphasized, and the student-doctor will be shown how to correctly find and assess the physical abnormalities in question. If the senior clinician revises the list of differential diagnoses and the diagnostic testing plan, the reasons will be explained to the student-doctor.

This is one of the most valuable interactions in terms of potential learning for the student-doctor. When a senior clinician helps you reason your way through what is typically the most difficult part of any medical case – the initial case presentation and workup– you begin to synthesize everything you learned in the classroom and merge it with the skills you'll need to apply your knowledge in the real world. This is how you will gradually learn to independently navigate the labyrinth of medical problem solving, client communication and patient care. Thinking your way through initial case presentation and workup under direct mentorship is the essence of practicing to practice medicine.

Once in a while it might actually happen just as I've described. More often though, you'll probably have to make your initial presentation standing in a busy hospital hallway while three other people vie for the senior clinician's attention with more pressing matters.

"Doctor Jones, they're still waiting for you in radiology. Doctor Smith needs to discuss his findings with you."

"Doctor Jones, Fluffy in the ICU is having breakthrough seizures. Do you want to increase her dose of phenobarbital or add another medication?"

"Doctor Jones, they're still waiting on you for that GI consult. Dr. White says you were supposed to be there ten minutes ago."

The need to be practical rather than perfect in a medical environment is always present. The senior clinician has many other responsibilities, and will often have to take shorts cuts, abbreviating the interaction with the student-doctor for the sake of his patients, and to keep the hospital running. On many days, senior clinicians, as much as they want to, simply won't be able to dedicate large blocks of time to thoroughly analyze and gently guide the student-doctor's thought processes.

Fourth year veterinary students are time pressured as well. Theoretically, after getting an initial history and performing an exam, you're supposed to find a quiet place to think so you can adequately prepare a cogent presentation. But, having used up all your allotted time filling out those persnickety forms, even at the expense of doing a thorough physical exam, you'll often have to present a poorly reasoned and incomplete plan.

"Hmmmm," the senior clinician may say, avoiding the urge to chastise you for not being more thorough. "Well... let's go take a look." And they'll be off, back to the exam room to do everything you did, only correctly and faster. Your duty then will be to chase them into the room, observe, and then chase them back out of the room as they dictate their diagnostic plan, which it will be your responsibility to transcribe onto more forms. Before you have the chance to ask them even one of the hundreds of questions flying helter-skelter through your brain like a colony of rabid bats, they'll already be on their way to one of the ten places they were supposed to be five minutes ago.

Passive Versus Proactive:
The Hospital Versus Your Brain

The first three years of veterinary school consist mostly of passive learning. You sit in a classroom, professors talk at you all day and give you notes to read. You study their notes, then you take their tests. You learn what your teachers tell you to learn. In contrast to those years in the classroom, it would seem that fourth year clinical rotations, where students work in a hospital setting, would consist of mostly active learning with student-doctors participating in the medical dialogue rather than merely receiving and regurgitating information. But the demands of the other roles you'll be expected to play will make it very tempting to passively go with the flow just to get through clinical rotations.

In the hurried chaos of the teaching hospital, you're going to want to avoid making waves - to avoid making things more complicated than they already are. You'll see the stress on your senior clinician's face and you'll just want to stay out of her way. This won't be difficult because, as I've already described, you'll have plenty of other work to keep you busy.

Even though there will be teaching and medical rounds, or discussion sessions, throughout each week, these are not adequate substitutes for working up real cases with direct mentorship. Rounds are helpful for learning medicine, but they're not the best method for teaching you how to practice medicine.

So here's the challenge of choosing to proactively practice practicing medicine: Your clinical education will consist of two separate, overlapping and competing forces. One force is the hospital, and in addition to the demands it places on your senior clinicians, it also includes your responsibilities as Master of Scutwork, Veterinary Assistant and Technician, and Laborer. The other force is your brain, and what takes place in your brain as you fulfill your other hospital duties. The quality of your clinical education will depend on whether you succumb to the temptation to passively perform, or choose instead to proactively exercise your brain despite the fatigue in your body.

Passively performing requires only that you show up every day on time, follow directions, fill out the forms, administer patient treatments, and appear to be doing your best when the doctors ask you questions in teaching and medical rounds. In this scenario, what you do with your brain can be limited to preparing to answer directed questions about specific medical topics that you'll often be told about ahead of time.

For example, on a Tuesday night of your ophthal-mology rotation you might be told that the next day's teaching rounds will be on the subject of "Neuroophthalmic Testing." A typical question you might get asked on Wednesday is, "What would you expect to see in an animal with right sided pre-chiasmic pathology if you performed a swinging flashlight test?" You won't fail out of fourth year if you get these questions wrong once in a while, or even pretty often, but you should be able to answer these questions correctly just by reading the section in your ophthalmology textbook called "Neuroophthalmic Testing."

Yet, answering questions like this is not practicing to practice medicine, and being able to answer these questions correctly is no indication that you're ready to practice independently. In the real world, the question would look more like this: A woman brings her dog to see you because his right eye looks "wrong." The entire globe of the dog's right eye appears abnormally enlarged, the cornea is cloudy and the sclera or "white of the eye" is covered in engorged blood vessels. Now what?

Being able to comprehensively respond to that question (and about a million more like it) is what you need to be able to do as a practicing veterinarian. By 'comprehensively respond,' I mean: What do you do next? And what are the next eight things you do after that? What do you ask your support staff to do? What do you tell the owner? Unlike the predictable, directed questions on specific medical topics you'll be asked in medical and teaching rounds, and the helpful prompts you can expect to receive from both the senior clinicians and your classmates, practicing in the real world consists of being presented with a sick animal, asking yourself "now what?" and having no one else there to help you answer that question.

This is why the student-doctor's interaction with the senior clinician is so crucial at the beginning of each case during your clinical rotations. These are the opportunities for you to try to answer those potentially paralyzing, big, gaping "now-what's" while someone else is there to help you. The more often you get to do this as a student-doctor, the better off you'll be as a real doctor after you graduate. If the forces of the hospital make your senior clinicians too busy to thoroughly mentor you through initial case presentations and workups, practicing to practice medicine will have to take place in your brain.

Cases will progress without your medical input in the hospital. The real doctors will see to this. Diagnostic tests will be conducted to either rule-in or rule-out various possible diagnoses until a final diagnosis is reached or all testing options have been exhausted. The doctors will develop a treatment plan. Changes to the treatment plan will be made by the doctors based on the patient's clinical response, and the doctors will order additional or ongoing testing as they deem warranted. You need only pay attention to the extent required to fill out the right forms, perform the correct treatments, accurately describe and update the case in the patient's daily medical record, and communicate with the pet's owner.

Your hospital responsibilities may require some understanding of medicine, but they do not require an understanding of how to practice medicine. For that you need to run each case separately in your brain, imagining yourself as the doctor in charge. Begin by developing your list of differential diagnoses and corresponding diagnostic testing plan as if the patient's life depended on you, rather than hurriedly throwing some ideas together knowing someone else is going to do the "real thinking." If your senior clinicians are juggling too many balls to hold your hand while new cases are being worked up, make mental notes of the key differences between your patient histories and the histories obtained by the senior clinicians, between your physical findings and those of your senior clinicians, between your lists of differential diagnoses and theirs, between your initial diagnostic plans and theirs.

While you're performing the scutwork of filling out multitudinous hospital forms for the diagnostic tests the doctors order, ask yourself why they might be suspecting different diseases than you are, and why they might be ordering different tests than you would. If the doctors found something on physical exam that you missed, while you're placing an IV catheter and starting IV fluids on the patient, repeat your physical exam, and try to find what they found. If the doctors were able to obtain key information from the owner that was not revealed when you were getting the patient history, while you're headed over to radiology to drop off an imaging request, ponder how you might have worded your questions differently to get a more accurate history. If your ruminations on these discrepancies produce no epiphanies, position yourself as necessary to intercept your senior clinicians before they leave the hospital for the night and directly ask them to help you understand the faults in your clinical reasoning, and to demonstrate the correct physical exam techniques required to identify any physical abnormalities in question.

I understand the will power this will require. You're going to be tired after your long, busy days and you will still have many duties to perform before you can go home. I also understand the courage this will require. Doctors can be intimidating, especially after they've had a long, busy day. And I certainly understand most students would prefer not to openly reveal the gaps in their understanding or the deficits in their abilities, especially to the doctors evaluating their performance on a rotation. But senior clinicians don't expect fourth year veterinary students to be perfect (even though they may sometimes act as if they do). What they want to see, more than anything, is evidence that you care, that you're thinking deeply and working hard to improve your knowledge and skills.

As cases progress from initial presentation to final diagnoses, there will many additional opportunities for you to choose to proactively exercise your brain. While the senior clinicians are devising their treatment plans (such as IV fluid rates, IV or oral medications, feeding schedules, monitoring protocols, etcetera), imagine yourself as the final authority on the case and develop your own treatment plans, including making all the calculations for fluid rates and medication doses. Compare yours against the real treatment plans and try to figure out the reason for any differences.

If you don't understand why a doctor ordered a particular treatment, ask them for their rationale. When you pick up blood work results to deliver to the doctors, do your best to interpret them on your own and consider whether you would change the treatment or diagnostic plans based on those results and why or why not. Think about how best to communicate the blood work results to the pet's owner. If radiographs have been taken, try to interpret the images before reading the radiologist's report. If you are unable to come to the same conclusions as the radiologist, ask him to help you see what he saw.

You can go through these mental exercises on your classmate's cases as well. When you get the chance, ask your classmates how they would handle a case, interpret test results or decide on a treatment plan. Discussing medical cases with your fellow student-doctors is another piece of practicing to practice medicine. If you've ever worked at a multi-doctor practice, you've probably noticed the doctors conferring with each other on their cases. They're seeking alternative perspectives because they know, regardless of seniority or years of experience, there's always something to be learned from someone who thinks differently.

Despite the work the hospital needs you to perform, for you, the priority of clinical rotations is to practice practicing medicine – and this is the only chance you'll ever get. The only person who can ensure you get a top notch clinical education is you, so be proactive, be courageous, be bold. Don't be shy or embarrassed to give the wrong answer, or to admit you don't know something, or that you don't know how to do something.

You will still have so much to learn as a fourth year student. The only person in the hospital who will expect you to already know everything and to be perfect - is you. Don't let these irrational fears prevent you from exposing the gaps in your knowledge. That's how we learn . As a fourth year veterinary student, it will be okay to make mistakes in clinical reasoning. So make them. Make as many thinking errors as you possibly can. The more you make as a student-doctor, the less you'll make when the time comes to practice medicine as a real doctor in the real world.

External Rotations

At VMRCVM, small animal trackers were permitted three external rotations. We could go anywhere outside of the teaching hospital for these rotations, providing the administrators approved our choices. You'll also have the opportunity to choose some external rotations. Here's what I suggest:

If Practice is your Goal, Surgical Experience is a Must

I fulfilled one of my external rotations at a non-profit animal shelter in Roanoke, VA called Angels of Assisi, where the bulk of my time was spent performing sterilization surgeries. For three straight weeks, I performed ovariohysterectomies and neuters on dogs and cats. As soon as I finished one surgery, a technician would carry the post-op patient to the recovery area and another technician would place a newly prepped, intubated and anesthetized patient on the operating table for me.

For hours at a time, I stood in the same spot behind that operating table. The shelter director was simultaneously performing surgeries on the adjacent table in the same surgical suite, and I could call on her whenever I needed guidance. I developed an intuition for handling living tissue, I improved my skills at correctly holding and maneuvering surgical instruments, became more adept at maintaining sterility, and dramatically improved the quality and speed of my suturing.

A couple months later, during my ophthalmology rotation, the ophthalmology resident rewarded me for shining in teaching rounds by allowing me to perform an enucleation. A dog with end stage glaucoma in one eye was having the eye removed as a palliative measure. The resident, who was still learning himself, could have used the opportunity to further his own surgical skills, but instead graciously gave me the gift of performing the operation under his supervision. One of the comments he made on my evaluation after the end of that rotation was, "Your surgical skills are truly a breath of fresh air." That meant so much to me that I saved his evaluation and still have it today, but it was the surgical experience I gained on the spay/neuter rotation that enabled me to impress him.

Before my rotation at Angels of Assissi, my surgical training had consisted of one canine neuter, one canine ovariohysterectomy, one feline ovariohysterectomy (all the animals being sterilized had come from local shelters), and a dental lab where my classmates and I practiced tooth extraction on a cadaver head (I extracted one mandibular canine). In each of these cases, I had to share practicing these procedures with three or four other students. In the sterilization procedures, only one student got to be the surgeon. The other students just assisted by handing instruments to the student performing the surgery or by keeping the long line of suture out of his way. Sometimes all you got to do was monitor anesthesia.

In the past, veterinary students were able to gain much more surgical experience during their clinical rotations. One reason is that purpose bred lab animals, usually beagles, were used for students to practice multiple surgeries (ovariohysterectomies, neuters, gastrotomies, enterotomies, resection and anastomoses, liver biopsies, splenectomies, etcetera) and then euthanized while under anesthesia during the final surgery of the semester. My friend, Dr. Campbell , went to vet school in the Caribbean many years ago and he told me of a goat that he and his classmates performed multiple surgeries on.

Throughout the semester, Dr. Campbell and his classmates were in charge of caring for this goat and they grew quite fond of him. They named the goat Frey. When Dr. Campbell described how after each surgery, Frey grew observably weaker and more depressed, and then how he had to euthanize Frey after the last surgery, Dr. Campbell's eyes filled with tears and his voice became choked with emotion. Nine years later, he still carried a tremendous burden of guilt and remorse for this.

I don't know whether terminal surgeries are still performed in some North American or Caribbean veterinary colleges today. My impression is that these are being phased out due increased awareness and public pressure. But at the time I was applying in 2007, some veterinary schools were still requiring them. I applied only to schools where I knew I wouldn't have to partake in these practices. I knew this meant I would graduate with little surgical experience, but I hoped after graduation to find mentors to help me become surgically proficient by operating on patients who actually needed surgery.

Greater protection for lab animals in the United States went into effect after 1979 when it became required for any U.S. federally funded institution using animals for research, testing or training to comply with policies developed by Institutional Animal Care and Use Committees (IACUC). These policies vary by school. IACUC at VMRCVM mandated that the laboratory beagles used by our school could only undergo so many procedures per day, and there was a limit to the total number of procedures that could be performed on any one animal.

None of these procedures, at least none involving veterinary students, were very invasive. They ranged from placing intravenous catheters to practicing bandaging techniques to performing endoscopies while the dogs were under anesthesia. After an animal had reached the limit of allowed procedures, rather than being euthanized, he was put up for adoption. My friend Chloe adopted one of the lab beagles. His name was Clooper, and after he left the laboratory, he enjoyed over seven years of happiness before he passed away from old age.

On the one hand, the dying tradition of terminal surgeries and the stricter protection for lab animals used in teaching are, in my opinion, positive signs that human consciousness is evolving for the better. On the other hand, veterinarians are graduating with insufficient surgical experience to confidently perform the procedures they are expected to perform. Additionally, the increase in the number of veterinary graduates pursuing internship and residency often means that, where a fourth year veterinary student might previously have been permitted to suture an incision closed after the board certified surgeon completed the difficult part of an operation, this opportunity is now more commonly granted to an intern or resident.

Whether a newly minted veterinarian ends up in a practice with good surgical mentoring or not is a mere matter of chance. Regardless of what the hiring manager or practice owner promises, it's impossible to know whether quality and reliable guidance will be provided when needed. Private hospitals, just like teaching hospitals, are busy places and it's often difficult for doctors to extract themselves from their own medical cases in order to coach a novice. For all these reasons, doing at least one of your external rotations at a spay/neuter facility is essential.

Get Some Good (Realistic) Day Practice Experience

A 2011 article entitled *Challenges and Opportunities Facing Medical Education* written by a human medical doctor states, "Approximately 80% of clinical education occurs in inpatient settings, yet 80-90% of medicine is practiced in the outpatient arena."[3] While I don't know of any available analogous statistics for veterinary medicine, my guess is they would be very similar. Most patients seen in a typical veterinary teaching hospital, whether they're there for an elective orthopedic procedure like a total hip replacement, or because they're being seen by internal medicine specialists for a serious illness, require hospitalization. This is inpatient medicine.

Teaching hospitals are specialty centers and have little in common, if anything, with day practices – which is where the majority of veterinary graduates will begin their careers. Veterinarians at day practice hospitals practice mostly, though not exclusively, outpatient medicine. When you go to see your regular doctor for a routine check up or for a cough or a urinary tract infection, and the doctor performs an exam, maybe runs a few basic diagnostic tests, prescribes some medication if needed, and sends you home – that's outpatient medicine.

On my Community Practice rotation, I only had the chance to see a handful of some common medical presentations like routine vaccine appointments and benign lumps and bumps. There was controversy when the school decided to open its Community Practice clinic. Critics stressed that the Community Practice service would be directly competing with local day practices, which the teaching hospital relied on for referrals. A backlash could result in a precipitous drop in referral cases. Therefore, VMRCVM's Community Practice services were not aggressively advertised to the surrounding community, and the caseload on this rotation was relatively low, at least while I was there.

Even in the best scenarios, I'm dubious that a general practice rotation inside a teaching hospital can give a student an accurate idea of what it's truly like to be a general practitioner in the real world. Veterinary teaching hospitals have resources day practice hospitals don't, such as MRIs and CT scanners, and are staffed with board certified specialists who can be consulted on the fly as you walk through the hallways.

The best place to do a general practice rotation is at a day practice hospital where you've previously worked as an assistant or technician, or where you know someone. If you already know someone at the practice, you're much more likely to have a positive and productive experience.

I fulfilled my second external rotation at the day practice where Dr. Campbell is an associate veterinarian. He developed a clever way of helping me gain experience in initial case work-up by making me responsible for every drop off. When pet owners are too busy to come in for an appointment, or if a pet owner wants their pet seen despite there being no open appointments, some clinics offer drop off services where the veterinarian will examine, diagnose and start treatment on a pet in the absence of the owner, provided the owner gives permission.

For my drop off patients, I would get the basic history

from the receptionist who admitted the pet, then perform my exam and present my findings, list of differential diagnoses, and recommended diagnostic tests to Dr. Campbell, who would mentor me through the case. I also got to participate in all of his interesting cases, as well as performing a neuter, a spay, and assisting him in a cryptorchid surgery (an operation to remove a testicle that failed to descend out of the abdomen into the scrotum).

The owner of the practice, a man with over thirty years of experience who had remained dedicated to keeping abreast with current medical protocols, also involved me in his interesting cases and went out of his way to mentor me. The support staff at this hospital were welcoming and helpful. I gained some great training as well as some much needed confidence thanks to all of them.

Positive as that experience was however, there were two important missing components. Firstly, doctors and student-doctors alike get excited about interesting medical cases rather than the hum-drum and common problems like skin or ear infections. Because of this understandable bias, I got to participate when patients presented with exotic things like immune mediated thrombocytopenia or transitional cell carcinoma, but I gained no experience in diagnosing or treating run of the mill medical conditions. You need to make sure you get to see a representative sample of medical cases at the day practice, not just the interesting ones, so tell the staff you're interested in participating in the kinds of cases they most commonly see.

Secondly, neither my Community Practice rotation nor my rotation at Dr. Campbell's practice gave me any appreciation for the most daunting challenge of being a general practitioner: Being bound to a rigid appointment schedule that allots every patient the same limited number of minutes while reality plays you like a contestant on a crapshoot television game show.

"Yes, ladies and gentlemen! Here we have our lovely contestant, Dr. April Kung, all the way from Flagstaff, Arizona, to play a round of *What's Really Behind that Door?* Dr. Kung, welcome to the show! I have in my notes here that you prefer to be called Dr. K. Is that right?"

"Yes, Dave, thank you. A lot of people ask how to pronounce my last name. I tell them it's like Kung-fu, but without the fu. After saying that the first hundred times, it's gotten pretty old for me."

"Hah ha, yes, I can see how you might get tired of saying that. Dr. K it is! So, Dr. K, are you feeling lucky today?"

"Well, Dave, I'm hoping to be lucky."

"Well said, Dr. K! Indeed, can any of us do anything but hope? Well, let's see what the cards have in store for you, shall we? Dr. K, could you please read for me what it says on the schedule for 1:40pm?"

"It says, 'New Puppy Exam,' Dave."

"Fantastic! New puppy exam! That sounds promising! After all, who doesn't love puppies? Don't you just love puppies, Dr. K?"

"Yes, Dave. I do love puppies. I love puppies very much."

"Alright then, Dr. K! Let's see if Lady Luck is with you today. Will you choose to perform your new puppy exam in the room behind Door Number One or Door Number Two? And remember! Regardless of which door you choose, you only have twenty minutes to complete this appointment in order to stay on schedule and keep everyone happy! Nobody likes it when the doctor's running late! Am I right?

"Right, Dave."

"Are you ready?"

"Yes, Dave. I'm ready. I've always had better luck with odd numbers so I'm going to go for Door Number One."

"Door Number One, ladies and gentlemen! Will it be the happy, healthy puppy wagging his tail and giving lots of puppy kisses who just needs his first distemper-parvo vaccine and belongs to polite and responsible pet owners? Let's see! Hey, pretty lady in the sparkly dress, please open Door Number One!"

Door number one opens. Sad trombone side effect: "Wah, wah, wah!"

"Oh! I'm so sorry Dr. K! Behind Door Number One we have a very lethargic and severely anemic puppy covered in fleas whose owners paid "a lot of money" for him from a disreputable breeder. They don't have any money left and are going to be very angry with you when you refuse to vaccinate him, and tell them their puppy needs an expensive blood transfusion instead! Tough luck, Dr. K! Better luck next time. Now get hopping! The clock is ticking!"

My suggestion for learning how to practice medicine against a clock is that you request to follow several different doctors, one per day, all day, for every single appointment. Do this for the first three to four days, if there are enough doctors to choose from. Following can be extremely boring without a clear objective in mind, but you're going to know exactly what to focus on. You're going to watch the clock.

When you're the doctor, you will be solely responsible for time management for both you and your support staff. How good you are at it will determine whether you get home in time for dinner most nights or spend your evenings writing records and making client callbacks alone in the clinic long after everyone else has gone home. So, while you're following, watch how each doctor handles his or her time and directs the support staff.

Know how long the appointments are and note what the doctors do and how they react when unexpected delays occur. If a client is being especially talkative, how does the doctor politely cut short the conversation? If the technicians are unable to get a blood sample for a heartworm test, observe whether the doctor is paying attention to this and whether she intervenes in order to keep the appointment on schedule.

How effectively do the different doctors use the support staff? Do they fill their own prescriptions? Run their own blood work? Read urinalyses and perform cytology themselves? If an appointment is taking longer than the time allotted, how does the doctor manage the completion of that appointment with the demands of the new appointment? Does Dr. X let his clients know when there's a delay? How does Dr. Y communicate with the front desk staff if she starts running behind? Is Dr. Z writing medical records between appointments or just jotting down some notes in order to complete his records at the end of the day? How do the different doctors manage to fit in client callbacks and requests for prescription refills in between their appointments?

You want to learn how different doctors manage multiple, competing and often unexpected demands against the clock. Some will be better at it than others, but if you pay close attention, you can learn something useful from all of them. If you have the opportunity to have lunch with the doctors, ask them for their best advice on time management from a GP's perspective. If you have the opportunity to have lunch with the support staff, ask for their opinions on effective ways of keep appointments running on schedule.

After your first several days of following, the clinic may have its own ideas about how you should be spending your time. More likely though, there will be opportunities for you to proactively design your own learning experience. You could easily spend the entire rotation being a wall flower if you just passively go with the flow, especially if you're at a clinic where you don't know anyone. It may be tempting just to take a break from all the responsibilities awaiting you back at the teaching hospital, but I urge you to take advantage of this temporary reprieve from teaching hospital duties to immerse yourself in the role of student-doctor.

Ask to read fecals, urinalyses, blood smears and ear and skin cytology under either doctor or technician supervision. Get good at those things. Ask the support staff if they would be willing to help you practice your time management skills and see if you can come up with a creative plan together to get you the practice you need at managing a team under a time limit without disrupting the actual hospital schedule.

Ask if you can perform spays or neuters or even laceration repairs or other simple procedures under doctor supervision. Ask to be responsible for seeing drop-offs and working up those cases under the mentorship of the hospital doctors. If you get to be in charge of drop off-cases, notice how long it takes you to work up cases. Where are you stumbling and losing the most time? To use a favorite chemistry saying, what's the rate limiting step? What feels most awkward? Is it physical exams? Is it getting histories? Is it coming up with differential diagnoses? Or designing diagnostic plans? Once you identify where you struggle, you can try different approaches to improve your efficacy and efficiency in those areas. You can also ask the doctors for specific recommendations on how to improve in those areas.

Do a Rotation at a (Recommended) Emergency Hospital

My third and last external rotation was at a specialty/ER hospital near Richmond, VA. I was very excited about the prospect of spending three straight weeks on overnight emergency duty with an experienced ER veterinarian, but I had made the mistake of not asking the administrators at my hospital for recommendations on where to do an ER rotation. Students complete evaluations on all their external rotations so future students can have some guidance as they make their external rotation selections. I should have availed myself of that resource.

The seasoned ER veterinarian at the emergency hospital I chose for my rotation was not happy to have me there. While she begrudgingly allowed me to follow her into exam rooms as she saw emergency appointments, she did not include me as she worked through her cases. She never invited me to round on the hospitalized patients with her, and I stood awkwardly at the technician station watching from a distance.

Most of the time, this ER vet acted like I was a piece of gum stuck to the bottom of her shoe. She wasn't just rude and impatient with me. She was rude and impatient with clients as well. I remember watching a distressed owner with his beloved Addisonian dog as he explained the unexpected life events that had prevented him from getting the monthly injection his dog needed from his regular veterinarian, which is why he came to the ER. The ER vet focused intently on picking the dirt from under her fingernails as the man talked. What this ER vet wanted, more than anything, was to finish all her work as fast as possible so she could go upstairs to the doctors' office and read mystery novels.

Luckily, a first year intern who had earned her DVM from the veterinary college in North Carolina, was on overnights three nights a week. I looked forward to the nights I would spend with her even more than I dreaded the nights I would spend with the other ER vet. This intern talked to me about every case and quizzed me about every medical issue represented in the hospital. Her enthusiasm for veterinary medicine and for teaching reinvigorated and inspired me. She gave me one of the best tips I ever received about practicing medicine, especially emergency medicine.

She showed me what she called her "bible." It was a hardbound, pocket notebook in which she had filled nearly every page with what she considered essential medical facts and formulae – some of which she learned in vet school (like the complicated protocol for treating diabetic ketoacidosis) – but most of which she learned after vet school, on her feet and in the weeds (like how to calculate the volume of fluid to use for an enema in a constipated cat). She didn't need to spend precious minutes looking these things up on the internet or in a textbook. They were right there in her pocket.

She advised me to make my own "medical bible," and I immediately set to work on it. I use it every day in the hospital. It saves me incalculable time. You should start making your own "medical bible" as a fourth year student too. Visit www.realize.vet/book2-resources for recommendations on how to do this, as well as to see pictures of some of the pages of my medical bible.

Knowing that this wonderful intern would be leaving halfway through my rotation, and unable to bear the thought of spending any more time with the other ER vet, I requested to switch to days and work with the Internal Medicine specialist for the remainder of my stay there. He, like the intern, loved to teach, and I learned an enormous amount from him in just a week and a half. In the real world (outside the teaching hospital) Internal Medicine specialists often see neurology cases and cancer cases and cardiology cases, as well as performing their own ultrasounds for lack of on-staff radiologists.

I still remember him as one of the most amazing doctors I've ever known. If I hadn't asked to switch to Internal Medicine, aside from the few nights I spent with the enthusiastic intern, I probably would have gained little from this rotation. This is another example of why it's important to be proactive as a fourth year student. If you're not getting what you think you need out of an external rotation, come up with a solution to fix the problem, and then... ask.

Even though I didn't get a lot of ER experience on that rotation, I did spend my first two and a half years out of vet school as an ER vet, so I can still tell you what to focus on in order to get the most out of an emergency medicine rotation. First of all, just like day practice, emergency medicine is also all about managing multiple, competing and unexpected demands against the clock. The difference is that there is no set schedule. Which patients get seen, when and for how long is 100% up to the ER vet.

In a lot of animal emergency hospitals, the ER vet is responsible for taking care of every animal that walks through the door, and also for every animal in the hospital. She will be balancing her attention, sometimes from minute to minute, between critically ill hospitalized patients and critically ill patients being carried into the hospital by hysterical owners. Sometimes she'll have to perform this balancing act during medical rounds, or even while she's in surgery.

Observe the doctor's demeanor during these stressful times. How does he handle the stress? Does he show it? What effect does that have on the support staff? Observe how he communicates with the support staff as medical priorities change. Does he ask a specific person to do a specific thing? Or does he tell everyone in the treatment area what needs to be done and leave it up to them? Which tactic seems to be more effective?

If the doctor is going to talk to owners in an exam room, does he tell his support staff where he's going and under what circumstances they should interrupt him? Does he direct his support staff to continually update owners who are waiting in the lobby? How does he handle angry or upset owners? Observe all of these things as if you will be in his shoes someday. You will. Even if you never practice emergency medicine, general practitioners have to handle emergencies too.

Secondly, if you do your ER rotation at a 24/7 ER hospital (recommended), during shift changes the outgoing doctor will brief the incoming doctor on every patient in the hospital. If at all possible, you should be present for these medical rounds, preferably at both the beginning of a shift (as the incoming doctor is learning all the important details about the hospitalized patients from the outgoing doctor), and at the end of a shift, (when the doctor you spent the shift with becomes the outgoing doctor and updates the next incoming doctor).

During these rounds, the doctors will discuss radiographs, blood work, medications, fluid therapy regimens, as well as the clinical status and prognosis for each patient. You'll get to watch them collaborate on and reason through complex medical issues. For a student-doctor, there's no better wall in the world to be a fly on than that of an emergency hospital during doctor rounds. Lengthy, detailed exchanges between doctors on multiple sick patients is not something you're likely to get to observe in any other setting.

Lastly, the ER technicians will probably also have their own medical rounds. If you can, I highly recommend you observe those as well. Emergency veterinary technicians are a special breed. They are typically very knowledge-able and highly skilled. I learned a lot from the ER technicians I worked with, and you will too if you pay attention.

Your Evaluations: To Read or Not to Read?

Clinical rotations are probably going to be the hardest part of veterinary school. You will experience high levels of physical, mental and psychological stress as you navigate the ever changing landscape of medical disciplines, doctors and support staff. At the end of each rotation, you will receive a written evaluation on your performance. Sometimes you're going to feel unfairly judged. Sometimes, after you've worked really hard on a rotation and you're expecting a great evaluation, what you're going to read instead will deeply disappoint you. Good evaluations can boost your confidence and morale, but lackluster or poor evaluations have the potential to severely demoralize you.

My first and only disappointing evaluation was from my pathology rotation. I received a low score because one of my evaluators felt I dressed inappropriately. We wore coveralls every day! Even though I knew this criticism was unfounded and unfair, it hit me very hard, and it hurt. It sucked all the energy out of my body and left me feeling like a deflated blue balloon that got thrown on the floor and was now covered with dirty footprints.

Want to know how I ensured it was my *only* disappointing evaluation? I stopped reading my evaluations after that. I recognized my susceptibility to negative feedback was heightened due to the stress of fourth year. I couldn't afford to let the subjective, hurried opinions of interns, residents and senior clinician's rob me of what little enthusiasm I was able to muster when I was already chronically exhausted. I knew that if I failed a rotation, someone from the administrative office would tell me. As long as that didn't happen, I was just going to go on doing the best I could, and never mind what was written in those evaluations.

If you do get a disappointing evaluation as a fourth year student, unless you've failed the rotation, just take it with a grain of salt. Remember, the people evaluating you are very busy and under a lot of stress themselves. Many of them will not have spent enough time with you one-on-one to accurately assess you, but it will be part of their job to do so. They may write something without thinking very hard, or when they're in a bad mood for some reason that has nothing to do with you. People are imperfect, and they have imperfect perceptions and opinions. If you recognize, like I did, that your susceptibility to negative feedback is heightened due to the stress of clinical rotations, just remember: You don't have to read your evaluations.

Cows and Pigs and Chickens, Oh My!

When I began veterinary school, I had every intention of becoming a mixed animal veterinarian. I wanted to be able to treat dogs and cats as well as horses, sheep, goats, pigs, cows, and chickens. I even dreamed of having my own little farm someday. It only took a couple weeks of medical lectures to change my mind. Learning about the differences in just the gastrointestinal tracts of these different species, I knew I would never feel comfortable practicing medicine on so many different kinds of animals.

I decided to become a small animal veterinarian instead, and from then on, focused most of my attention on learning about dogs and cats. I retained only as much information about horses, sheep, goats, pigs, cows, and chickens as I felt necessary to pass my exams, and eventually, the North American Veterinary Licensing

Examination (NAVLE), which is a generalized examination covering basic medical knowledge for all these species. I eagerly looked forward to the day when I would receive news that I'd passed this national exam, because I knew on that day, I would unceremoniously dump out of my brain everything I'd ever learned about animals I would never touch as a doctor, to make more room for the multiple encyclopedias worth of information I knew I still needed to learn about dogs and cats.

VMRCVM offered a tracking program, for which I will be forever grateful. As a small animal tracker, I was able to benefit from many elective classes that focused solely on companion animal medicine. I got to skip many classes that focused on food animal or equine medicine. However, courses that were a part of the core curriculum still required me to memorize such irrelevancies as how to identify different breeds of cattle or the recommended de-worming schedules for horses. I don't resent my veterinary school for this. They had to do it this way in order to prepare students to pass the NAVLE. You can't practice veterinary medicine on any species unless you pass the NAVLE, and the NAVLE asks you about every species you study in vet school.

Just as the core curriculum throughout the first three years of veterinary school required me to learn about species in which I had no medical interest, I couldn't escape the requirement of having to practice practicing medicine on these species as a fourth year veterinary student. Many of the core clinical rotations like Radiology, Anesthesia, Ophthalmology, and Pathology were not specific to dogs and cats. In those rotations my small animal clinical education was diluted, as my lecture based education had been, by having to divert my attention to things I would never need to know as a small animal veterinarian - like taking radiographs of horse knees, or sedating goats, or treating mammary gland infections in dairy cows, or how to perform a necropsy on a bloated bull that had been dead for several days.

My husband had two years of lectures in medical school, leaving two years for his medical school clinical rotations. After that, he spent three years as an Internal Medicine Resident. He had *five years* to practice practicing medicine on one species! By contrast, I got one year to practice practicing medicine on eight species. Even though I knew I was getting off easy thanks to VMRCVM's tracking program, and it could certainly have been worse, I was still quite displeased to learn that, in addition to core rotations being diluted with large animals, I also had to complete two rotations that focused strictly on large animals. If you'd have asked me at the time, that was two too many.

Rectal Palpations

The weeks I spent on my large animal rotations endowed me with some uniquely vivid memories that will never fade. There were horses and occasionally a few cows or goats to take care of in the hospital, but mainly there were farm calls at all hours of the day or night. Both my large animal rotations took place in the winter.

Winter in Virginia gets nowhere near as cold as winter where I grew up in Chicago, but when you can see the bright side of having to insert your arm into the warm rectum of a milk cow while her rectal muscle contractions squeeze out a continuous stream of steaming, loose manure that cascades over your shoulder and falls onto your feet with a sound that is a surprising combination of both a "plop" and a "splash" – you know it's just too darn cold outside.

The point of rectal palpations, contrary to the name, is not typically to palpate (examine by touch) the rectum, but to find and palpate the ovaries through the rectal wall. Experts can tell what stage of the breeding cycle a cow is in by what the ovary feels like. To this day I continue to puzzle over what law of physics or temperature differentials might explain why every time I stuck my arm in a cow's rectum, the yellow plastic sleeve I wore expanded inside with so much air that the rectum became a cavernous space and the mucosal surface became plasticized.

Honestly, it was not wholly unpleasant to pat the inside of those large plasticized rectums, but the rectal walls were substantially less pliable under these conditions, and I was unable to feel even prominent intra-abdominal structures, much less a little ovary about half the size of the palm of my hand. The large animal veterinarians would ask me, as I flopped my hand about inside these secret plastic caves, whether I had found the ovary. All of my classmates claimed to have found ovaries. After a while I succumbed to peer pressure and lied that yes, I had. But the truth is, of the dozens and dozens of rectal palpations I performed during my large animal rotations, I never found an ovary. If the same thing happens to you, I wouldn't sweat it.

Cryptospoidiosis

Cryptosporidiosis is a zoonotic illness (meaning it's transmissible between humans and other animal species) that causes frequent, watery diarrhea and painful abdominal cramps. Veterinary students learn to fear this parasitic infection in their early years of school when they hear horror stories from fourth year students who contracted this illness on their large animal rotations. In vet school, typically the infectious organisms come from sick calves. I was determined to avoid this illness at all costs. When one of our large animal professors offered the opportunity to perform a physical exam on a pathetic looking, lethargic calf whose coat was encrusted with dried diarrhea, I declined. One of my classmates, however, jumped at the chance. I made the mistake of sharing my water bottle with him later that day. He came down with symptoms of Cryptosporidiosis a few days later, and the day after that, I did too.

My symptoms peaked on the day I had to take a long road trip with two of my classmates and one large animal veterinarian to a distant dairy farm where we would spend the entire day – you guessed it – performing rectal palpations. During the three hour ride, we had to make six urgent bathroom stops because of me. Once we arrived, I spent half the day in the farmhands' outhouse and the other half sitting on the cold ground cradling my head in my hands. No matter how much water I drank, I remained dehydrated, and this resulted in a debilitating headache. On the bright side, I didn't have to stick my arm into any cow rectums that day.

You will learn in your lectures on infectious disease that the severity and duration of one's symptoms is affected, in part, by the number of infectious organisms one is exposed to. You can think of this quantity of infectious organisms sort of like a dose. The larger the number of organisms, the greater the dose. Since my exposure to Cryptosporidium was indirect (via the water bottle I shared with my classmate), my dose was low and my symptoms resolved after only a few days. My gung-ho classmate was significantly sicker than I and his symptoms lasted for two weeks because of the enormous dose of Cryptosporidium he got from examining that poor, sick calf. The moral of this story is firstly, if given the choice, don't touch any calves with diarrhea, and secondly, never share any eating or drinking paraphernalia with anyone on a large animal rotation. Ever.

Are You Sure You Don't Want to be a Large Animal Veterinarian?

One of my large animal professors, Dr. Whittier, was a spry man of about seventy. He was always kind but it was clear he wasn't thrilled with the changes he was seeing in his vocation. I can empathize with his chagrin, as over the decades, he witnessed the transition of veterinary medicine from a mostly male profession focused on farm animals to an industry quickly becoming female dominated and concentrated on house pets. He was a bit old-fashioned, but he was a good man and I never detected any true sexism. In fact, he was endlessly trying to turn every student who planned to practice small animal medicine, whether male or female, into large animal veterinarians.

I wouldn't be surprised if he never converted anyone. Not because he wasn't persuasive. He was really quite charming. But he was fighting a losing battle because people planning to go into small animal medicine have visions of themselves working indoors in a climate controlled environment, wearing nice clothes under a snow white lab coat, and forming emotional bonds with their patients. Convincing them to exchange that dream for a mostly outdoor job where the daily attire consists of coveralls and knee high rubber boots, and where patients are considered production units instead of beloved family members is an almost impossible sell.

I once had to go on an overnight assignment with Dr. Whittier to a beef cattle farm that was a half a day's drive away. The last time I had taken a road trip with Dr. Whittier, he talked to me for two straight hours about all the different cuts of beef and what qualities were used to grade them. Despite finding this impromptu lecture mildly interesting, there were about twenty other things I had wished to be doing instead. Having to converse about meat cuts for two hours left me drained even before we arrived to the farm where we had to vaccinate three hundred calves. Now I was going to ride in a truck with him for an entire day, stay overnight, and spend the following day performing breeding soundness exams on a herd of *four hundred fifty* bulls. I was indescribably relieved when I heard my friend Renee (also a small animal tracker) and a 6'4" tall male student named Chris would also be coming along. Chris was visiting from the veterinary school at the University of Pennsylvania and – and thank goodness - he wanted to be a large animal veterinarian. I know Dr. Whittier was as relieved to have Chris along as I was.

The following morning, as Dr. Whittier was packing supplies into the mobile veterinary truck, I got to witness a most marvelous juxtaposition: A manly-man large animal veterinarian having to confront the girly-girl proclivities of two small animal trackers. Renee and I, as girls are prone to do, had both stereotypically over packed, and Dr. Whittier was struggling to fit Renee's large suitcase into the vehicle's storage compartment. He was in the process of jumping on the metal flatbed storage door to get it to close over Renee's suitcase when Renee exclaimed, "Oh Dr. Whittier! Please be careful! I have face cream in that bag!"

During the six hour drive, Chris and Dr. Whittier talked happily in the front of the truck while Renee and I enjoyed being left to ourselves in the back. By the time we closed in on our final destination, the sky was moonless and dark. Dr. Whittier had previously informed me we would be sleeping in a barn and I was mentally preparing myself for the misery to come. Would there be electricity? Running water? A toilet? I don't know about Renee, but that's was why I over packed. My suitcase contained a quilt, a pillow, and - just in case the barn had electricity - an electric blanket. Much to my relief we spent that night at a hotel just a few miles from the farm. Chris and Dr. Whittier shared a room, and Renee and I shared another. While the four of us were having dinner together that night, I asked Dr. Whittier why we were staying at a hotel instead of a barn. He just smiled slyly and winked. Such was my perception of what it was really like to be a large animal veterinarian, it never occurred to me he might have been joking when he told me we would be sleeping in a barn.

Our work began the next morning before sunrise at 4am. We checked out of the hotel because Dr. Whittier was determined to drive back to campus and home that night, no matter how late it was by the time we finished. Dr. Whittier explained that the bulls were being corralled behind the barn in which we'd be working. The bulls would enter the barn in pairs from the back and would be funneled by metal gates into two side-by-side cattle chutes where we would catch them using the part of the chute called a headgate. As they walked forward through the chute, the headgate would be shut behind their heads, entrapping them at their necks and preventing them from moving forward or backward.

Once the first two bulls were restrained, Dr. Whittier measured the circumference of the first bull's scrotum and then inserted an electro-ejaculator probe into the bull's rectum. Several electrical charges were delivered through the probe to cause the bull to ejaculate. Chris and Dr. Whittier were to take turns measuring and electro ejaculating alternate bulls. My job was to collect the semen into a test tube as the bull was ejaculating. For this, I had to kneel on the cold, dirty, concrete floor of the barn and intently watch the tip of the bull's penis in order to correctly time the collection. Rachel's job was to record the scrotal circumference and the identifying number from the bull's ear tag.

After the semen was collected, Renee and I looked at a sample under a microscope to estimate a sperm count and to grade the overall motility of the sperm. Renee recorded this information and then used another semen sample to create a stained slide, which was labeled with the bull's tag number and stored in a slide box. Each of the four hundred fifty stained slides would be analyzed under a microscope later in the week to gauge the quality of the sperm based on their morphology. While Renee and I were performing our lab duties, Dr. Whittier and Chris released the first bull out the front of the barn, filled the chute with a third bull from the back of the barn, and set up the electro ejaculator next to the second bull who was still restrained in the other chute.

When Renee and I were done with the lab work on the first sample, we took our positions so the whole process could be repeated on the second bull. This seemingly endless parade of angry, loudly vocalizing bulls went on until noon, when we took a short lunch, then continued until we were down to just a few remaining bulls around 8pm. The sun had long since set and the barn was cold, damp and dark. We were working by the dim light that trickled down from a handful of 60 watt bulbs in the barn's ceiling twelve feet over our heads. We'd been working for over fifteen hours.

My face and hands were filthy. My fingers were numb. I had sticky, dried bull semen in my hair, on my neck and all over the front of my coveralls. Several large, gooey globules of the stuff had found their way to the crevices of my left ear.

Perhaps Dr. Whittier had been impressed by how hard I worked despite being a girly-girl future small animal vet, or perhaps he just felt sorry for me. Whatever the reason, he decided to give me the honor of performing a vasectomy on one of the remaining bulls. The procedure would turn this bull into a "teaser," and he would be used to identify cows who are ready to breed. The teaser may mount them, he just can't impregnate them. While Chris and Rachel used the first chute to continue working on the last few bulls, Dr. Whittier and I positioned ourselves behind the bull in the second chute.

Both bulls were vocalizing so Dr. Whittier had to shout instructions at me on how to inject an epidural anesthetic while he gave a sedative. As these drugs were taking effect, Dr. Whittier injected a local pain blocking medication into the testicles and scrubbed the surgical site. I put on a pair of sterile gloves and Dr. Whittier handed me a scalpel. It was too dark for me to see clearly so Dr. Whittier aimed a pocket flashlight over my shoulder at the incision site. There were two incisions to be made, since our goal was to cut the vas deferens (the tube that carries sperm from the testicles to the urethra) for both testicles.

Dr. Whittier told me where to cut, how deep to cut and how long to make my cuts. As I made my incisions, the bull stirred. I was certain I was going to get kicked in the face, but instead the bull began sinking toward the filthy barn floor, taking his testicles and the open surgical wounds with him. The sedative was hitting him hard. Dr. Whittier walked to the front of the chute and clapped and yelled in the bull's face to shock him awake. The bull stood back up but his testicles had become covered in dirt, and I worried the surgical site would become contaminated.

Dr. Whittier returned to my side and shouted at me over the clanging, clattering sounds of the bull in the adjacent chute struggling against the metal restraints. He identified both vas deferens and instructed me to place two strangulating sutures around each, leaving an inch between them. I lacked the manual dexterity to comply because my fingers had gone numb from the cold long before we started the procedure. Dr. Whittier had to put on surgical gloves and perform this part of the operation. When he'd finished he had me transect both vas deferens between the two sets of double sutures. Once this was done, I was to suture both incisions closed in two separate layers.

The bull kept sinking to the ground as I tried to close the surgical wounds and Dr. Whittier had to repeatedly run to the front of the bull and yell in his face to wake him back up, taking the flashlight with him each time and leaving me to suture in the dark. Every time the bull started sinking, I had to track the downward movement of his testicles with my hands since the suture was attached to the skin of his scrotum and I was holding the suture. Dr. Whittier was also becoming progressively more interested in what Chris and Renee were doing instead of what I was doing. He was shouting directions at them as I continued trying to suture. Every time he spoke to Chris and Renee, the flashlight moved, and I would lose sight of the incision.

I tried my best to appear outwardly calm, but inwardly I was horrified. A vivid comparison flashed through my mind: The chaotic surgical procedure I was performing while exhausted beyond reason and covered in bull semen in this noisy, cold, dark, dirty, stinky barn – versus - the orderly ovariohysterectomy I'd previously performed on a twenty pound pug while listening to Mozart in the clean and brightly lit surgical suite of Dr. Campbell's hospital. After I tied the knot of the last suture, I closed my eyes and sighed. I was secretly thanking my lucky stars I was going to be a small animal veterinarian when Dr. Whittier exclaimed excitedly into my left ear, "ISN'T THIS BETTER THAN SMALL ANIMAL MEDICINE?!"

About a week later, Dr. Whittier bestowed another honor on me when he let me perform a standing cesarean section on a goat that was unable to deliver her baby naturally. A paravertebral pain block was administered as well as a localized pain block all along the tissues where the incision would be made. I was amazed how well it worked. That goat just stood there as if nothing were happening while I incised through her flank and into her uterus to extract her baby. I handed the kid to Dr. Whittier and he cleaned the amniotic fluid off and introduced him to his mother. Mother and kid nuzzled each other as I put my surgical experience from the shelter rotation to use to suture the surgical wound closed. Dr. Whittier exclaimed with pleasure, "I think April's done some needle work in her time!"

Old fashioned (but not sexist) comment aside - after all, Dr. Whittier let me perform two surgeries instead of granting those opportunities to my male classmates - I ended up with a wonderful sense of pride and accomplishment – and not just because of the surgeries. Though I had resented the time on my large animal rotations as depriving me of what I could have been learning about small animal medicine, in retrospect, my experiences on those rotations, and especially the times I had with Dr. Whittier, have become some of my fondest memories, as well as the source of many funny stories.

And even though he wasn't successful in converting me to large animal medicine, I wouldn't trade those memories for money or gold. Because, even though I may be a girly-girl, I survived large animal medicine rotations, and that means I can do anything. After you finish your large animal rotations, you'll feel that way too.

To Intern or Not to Intern?

At this time, except for the state of Oregon, veterinary school graduates are not required to do an internship before they can practice independently,[1] therefore unless Oregon is your destination after vet school or you plan to specialize, the choice is yours to pursue an internship or not. I did not. In addition to the fact that I think people are gross, not having to do an internship was one of the reasons I chose to become a DVM instead of an MD.

I started veterinary school when I was thirty-eight. When I was younger, like you probably are, I was all for picking up and living anywhere else in the world, just for the adventure. I spent seven years living in various countries in Asia Pacific. But the older you get, the more couches you own, and the more trouble it is to move. Life becomes more complicated.

By the time I graduated veterinary school, my father was in his seventies and had had a major stroke. He was paralyzed on the left side of his body and wheelchair bound. After vet school, I had to move back to Chicago to look after him.

Being an older student in veterinary school surrounded by mostly twenty-something classmates, I was envious. They were not yet burdened by the responsibilities, material possessions or even the rigid preferences and penchants for predictable routines that typically accompany middle age. They were unbound and had many more years in front of them than I. Most of them would start their careers as veterinarians long before they turned thirty.

I watched several of them fall in love (and sometimes out of love). I knew a few who travelled overseas during breaks and heard others planning future world travels. I knew I was being greedy. I had had my days to feast at the table of all possibilities, to sample every dish at my leisure knowing I could follow any whim as I selected from the menu. After all, when you're young and free, there's plenty of time before the kitchen closes to order something else if the first few entrées don't agree with you. The kitchen would remain open for my young vet school classmates for a long time after they graduated. They could afford to try many different options. But for me, the kitchen had closed.

If you're a straight arrow, still young and free by the time you finish veterinary school, my personal advice would be to take every advantage of your days to feast at the table of all possibilities. Do an internship, if you can, purely for the adventure and the excitement that comes from throwing yourself to the wind just to see what happens and where you end up.

It won't be a vacation. You will have to work long hours under intense pressure, but when you're young, you can do this and still enjoy the thrill that comes from pushing yourself to the limit. My guess is you'll discover how strong and amazing you actually are. That's the experience I had when I began my career in corporate advertising in Hong Kong at the age of twenty-five. For a pittance, I worked eighteen hour days, sometimes seven days a week, for weeks at a time, when there was an important campaign going on - and there was always an important campaign going on. It was hard, but also exhilarating, and no experience is more likely to spur exponential learning than intense immersion.

The AVMA Task Force on Veterinary Internships published an internship survey in the Journal of the American Veterinary Medical Association in late 2013. According to this survey, compared to respondents who had started practicing independently right after veterinary school, "significantly higher percentages of respondents who had participated in internships rated themselves as having become extremely or very competent" in general and advanced clinical skills, as well as communication skills, and almost 95% of those who had completed internships "felt they were better veterinarians because of their internship experience."[10]

This isn't surprising to me. Yes, retrospectively I recognize the need for fourth year veterinary students to practice the skills of veterinary assistants and technicians, however, the other side of that coin is that fourth year veterinary students get few *real* opportunities to actually practice practicing medicine. Imagining yourself as the real doctor as you reason through cases will help, but it is nowhere near as valuable as actually getting the be the doctor while still being supervised by senior clinicians – to really "practice with a net."

The internship survey also found that the average time "worked with supervision each week was significantly greater for respondents who entered internships than for those who entered clinical practice."[10] I am unaware of any studies comparing the emotional health of veterinarians who started independent practice after an internship against those who began practicing independently immediately after graduating, but I'd wager those who complete internships before practicing independently would enjoy better mental and emotional health.

Some percentage of poor patient outcomes are inevitable in either scenario, but the vast burden of the emotional toll of a poor outcome will always fall on the doctor in charge. The intern has one additional year of being at least partially shielded from the emotional tolls or poor patient outcomes. As well, the intern gains experience that will likely decrease their propensity for making medical errors when they do begin to practice without a net.

This being said, and despite all my romanticizing, it's still important to weigh the costs and the risks of pursuing a veterinary internship. In a spring of 2012 issue of the Journal of the American Veterinary Medical Association, an article entitled, "A call for internship quality control," estimated that based on the difference between average starting salaries of new veterinary graduates going straight into clinical practice, and those of veterinary interns, and combining that dollar amount difference with the accrual of interest on the average student loan during internship year, a veterinary internship was estimated to cost about $50,000. Furthermore, unlike veterinary residencies which lead to specialization, internships do not lead to higher salaries later.

The authors concluded that, fiscally speaking, veterinary internships are not worth what they cost, and therefore the "intangible benefits of an internship must be high for the internship to be considered time and money well spent."[5] In other words, an internship has to provide high quality teaching to justify its financial cost. But here's the problem: In human medicine, both internships and residencies are accredited by the Accreditation Council for Graduate Medical Education (ACGME). While there are accreditation agencies for veterinary residencies, none exist for veterinary internships. This means there are no universally enforced minimum standards for the quality of veterinary internships.[5] There are some great veterinary internships out there. But there are some really terrible ones too. So, caveat emptor. If you plan on doing a veterinary internship because you want a year practicing with a net, make sure you spend that $50,000 wisely. Do your homework. Visit www.realize.vet/book2-resources for some tips on how to select an internship.

In Closing

When you get your first acceptance letter for veterinary school, you're going to experience such elation. And you should. Getting into veterinary school is an amazing accomplishment for which you should be extremely proud. When you start veterinary school, you're going to feel incredibly excited and optimistic about your future. And you should. You'll be embarking on an adventure that so many long to experience but never will. And it truly is an amazing adventure. Despite the hardships, I still look back on veterinary school as one of the best and most exciting experiences of my life.

However, you should also be well prepared for the reality of how difficult a period this is going to be. Although I mention the importance of maintaining your health only briefly in this book, I hope the rest of the book gives a clear idea of the importance of self-care as you face the challenges of veterinary school. According to a 2008 study, 32% of first year veterinary students met the criteria for clinical depression.[7] Rates of depression in veterinary students have been shown to increase in clinical rotations.[6] This is not how I want you to begin your career as a veterinarian.

My deepest hope is that the information provided in this book will empower you with the advanced knowledge necessary to step into your role as a veterinary student ready for the challenges, rather than being blindsided and overwhelmed by them. You can get through it. You will get through it. Just please remember to take care of yourself along the way. Use the tools I gave you in Book 1. And do your best to take care of your classmates too. Foster kinship, not competition. For four hard years, the other hundred or so people in your class are going to face the same challenges and hardships as you. Please try to support and look out for each other.

For a list of recommended reading related to the topics in this book, go to www.realize.vet/book2–resources

 If you found this book helpful, I'd really appreciate if you would leave a positive review where you purchased it online.

Thank you for giving me the privilege of sharing what I know to enhance your experiences as you make the same journey to become a veterinarian that I made years ago.

If you have comments or suggestions for improving any of the books in this series, or if you have additional questions you would like to see addressed on my blog or on my podcast, please fill out the survey at www.realize.vet/survey

From the bottom of my heart, I wish you successful and magnificent future as a happy and healthy Doctor of Veterinary Medicine.

Kindest regards,
Dr. K
Flagstaff, Arizona

Index

1. Application for Oregon State Veterinary Medical License:
   http://www.oregon.gov/OVMEB/pdfs/Applicatio ns/Vet_App.pdf

2. Clance, Pauline Rose and Imes, Susanne. "The Imposter Phenomenon in High Achieving Women: Dynamics and Therapeutic Intervention." *Psychotherapy Theory, Research and Practice.* Volume 15, #3, Fall 1978.

3. Densen, Peter, MD. "Challenges and Opportunities Facing Medical Education." *Transactions of the American Clinical and Climatological Associatio.* 2011. Volume 122.

4. Duffy, Thomas P., MD. "The Flexnor Report - 100 Years Later." *Yale Journal of Biology and Medicine,* 84 (2011), pp.269-276.

5. Geller, John, DVM, et al. "A Call for Internship Quality Control." Journal *of the American*

Veterinary Medical Association. April 15, 2012. Volume 240, No. 8.

6. Larkin, Malinda. "The Hidden Curriculum." *JAVMA News*, May 15, 2017.

7. Larkin, Malinda. "The Toll it Takes to Earn a Veterinary Degree." *JAVMA News*, Dec. 15, 2014.

8. Ludmerer, Kenneth M., "The Internal Challenges to Medical Education." *Transactions of the American Clinical and Climatological Association,* VOL. 114, 2003.

9. Porter, Roy. *The Greatest Benefit to Mankind.* New York: W. W. Norton & Company, Inc., 1999.

10. Shepherd, Allison J., et al. "Veterinary Internship Survey, 2012." *of the American Veterinary Medical Association.* October 1, 2013. Volume 243, No. 7.

11. Weir, Kirsten. "Feel Like a Fraud?" The American Psychological Association, 2013.